Spare I

ABOUT THE AUTHOR

Paul Craddock is Honorary Senior Research Associate in the Division of Surgery and Interventional Science at UCL Medical School in London. His PhD explored how transplants have for centuries invited reflection on human identity, a subject on which he has also lectured internationally. *Spare Parts*, which won a Special Commendation from the Royal Society of Literature, is his first book.

Spare Parts

An Unexpected History of
Transplant Surgery

PAUL CRADDOCK

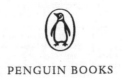

PENGUIN BOOKS

PENGUIN BOOKS

UK | USA | Canada | Ireland | Australia
India | New Zealand | South Africa

Penguin Books is part of the Penguin Random House group of companies
whose addresses can be found at global.penguinrandomhouse.com

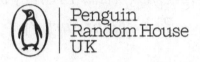

First published by Fig Tree 2021
Published in Penguin Books 2022
002

Copyright © Paul Craddock, 2021

The moral right of the author has been asserted

Printed and bound in Great Britain by Clays Ltd, Elcograf S.p.A.

The authorized representative in the EEA is Penguin Random House Ireland,
Morrison Chambers, 32 Nassau Street, Dublin D02 YH68

A CIP catalogue record for this book is available from the British Library

ISBN: 978–0–241–37026–1

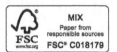

For Patricia

Contents

List of Illustrations

Prologue

The kidney bloomed, going from a miserable grey to many shades of vital red as blood rushed through its newly connected vessels. An organ that could seconds ago have been mistaken for discarded offal was now filled with life, resurrected and visibly claimed by a new body. This was my first time watching a kidney transplant.

I'd met the kind-eyed patient twenty minutes before he went under and watched as three scrubbed-up figures draped his body with green sheets. He disappeared under these by degrees like the Cheshire Cat fading into the landscape. But instead of a smile, we were left with a disembodied abdomen. As anonymous figures placed the last of the drapes, an auxiliary burst in with a trolley, pushing it up against the wall between a switched-off respirator and a rack of gleaming metal instruments. It was the donor kidney, lying on a bed of ice, monochrome and well trimmed with fat. Much like its intended recipient under the drapes, its life had been suspended. It resembled a calf's kidney past its sell-by date – an impression at odds with its true value. The desperately ill Mr Bhatti had received it as a gift from his brother, who was now recovering on a ward elsewhere in the hospital.

The two surgeons and their assistants stood either side of the abdomen, absorbed in the business of making their way through layers of skin, fat and muscle. Surgeons prefer diathermy for this job nowadays, burning rather than slicing the parts asunder. There is less bleeding this way but, until they break through into the cavity, the scorched flesh fills the operating theatre with the aroma of a Sunday barbecue. Once they'd finished severing the final bits of sinew, the pace slowed as the surgical team prepared the inner landscape of the abdomen, identifying, teasing out and labelling arteries, veins and the ureter. During these hours of intense concentration, my attention was drawn to the 'new' organ lying almost forlornly on its trolley. As time went by, blood leached out of it, its bed of ice slowly reddening.

I'd half expected the insistent beep of a heart monitor and steady hiss of a respirator to fill the room with urgency, but the machines keeping Mr Bhatti alive were silent. Crocs shuffled on the polished floor as one of the surgeons made his way over to the kidney and lifted it from its bed. He brushed away the flakes of red ice with the back of a gloved finger. Holding it aloft and cupping it in his hands, he then brought it to the operating table, where four more hands were ready to receive and stitch it in. A pause. The lead surgeon invited me up to the table to peer inside the cavity, hands behind my back so I wouldn't touch anything. Amongst the red anatomy, this lifeless grey mass looked diminished, limp and out of place. Three vessels connected it to the rest of the body, with tiny clamps temporarily stopping the flows of blood and urine. Before my eyes, the surgeon removed these devices and in a matter of seconds the kidney turned from grey to pink, then almost red. It seemed as if life itself had cascaded from one man's body into another's.

Everything about this experience suggested that transplantation was a decidedly modern concern. The theatre was crowded with complex machines, sophisticated instruments and digital displays. Chemical smells accompanied the aroma of burning human flesh. The procedure was a sterile, well-choreographed affair. But transplant surgery is far from an exclusively modern phenomenon, with a surprisingly long and rich history that stretches back as far as the Pyramids.

This story begins with the seemingly unremarkable skin graft – the first operation to move a body part from one place to another. Skin grafts would later become integral to working out the biological mechanism for tissue rejection, but they also are ancient transplants in their own right. The earliest reference to this kind of transfer was a skin-graft technique recorded in ancient India, mentioned in the Sushruta Samhita. This sacred book – an Ayurvedic text from the sixth century BC that also instructs surgeons on how to perform cataract surgery and what would later be called a caesarean section – explains how to take the skin from a person's forehead and shape it into a replacement for a lost nose. It's the earliest technical description of a transplant, and since the Samhita is a record of the surgery its writers considered to be already traditional, the technique itself is likely to be far older. There's a note at the end of the description, too, hinting at its pedigree: only those who could master skin grafting were considered sufficiently skilled to treat a king.

Although surgeons almost certainly performed rudimentary skin grafts for millennia, records of *any* transplants are sketchy to non-existent before the sixteenth century. But long before this, they featured in myths. Some of these provide an insight into the continued relevance and cultural significance of transplants, and would even come to influence the way many people viewed real-life transplant surgery in the centuries to come. In 1680, for instance, Chinese writer Pu Songling recorded the story 'Judge Lu', which follows the blossoming friendship between a brave but stupid man called Zhu Erh-Tan and the eponymous judge of the underworld. One day Zhu's friends convinced him to steal a likeness of the judge from the local temple. He got drunk, tottered off to the temple and stumbled back with the judge's full-size image, complete with green face and red beard. Before returning it, the drunken Zhu slurred an invitation for Judge Lu to join him for a glass of wine. No response. But the next night, there was a knock at his door. Zhu opened it to find the judge, risen from the underworld, standing before him. He immediately apologized for taking liberties with his image, fully expecting to lose his head for his insolence. Laughing off the misunderstanding, the judge reassured Zhu he'd come only to take him up on his offer of a drink.

After this, the odd pair got together every few days and became drinking companions. One day, Zhu went off to sleep, leaving the judge to drink alone. From deep in his slumber Zhu felt a stabbing pain in his chest and woke to find the judge sitting at the edge of his bed. His friend's hands were immersed in his chest, his fingers prodding around to find his heart. Though Zhu was terrified, Lu meant no harm. He was in fact performing an innocent heart transplant. Knowing his friend was stupid, and feeling sorry for him, he'd brought him a gift from the netherworld: a new heart – a clever one to replace the old stupid one, which he slapped onto the table as he tugged it out of Zhu's chest. Thanks to this new heart, Zhu was no longer stupid, and he became a great writer.

But the story doesn't end there. Zhu was naturally thankful for his transplant and asked whether the judge might similarly help his wife with *her* problem. Her figure was 'not bad', Zhu explained, but her face was ghastly. Might it be possible to switch her ugly head for a pretty one? Such a transplant would not threaten his wife's personality; the change would be merely cosmetic (in China at that time the 'person' supposedly resided in the heart – hence Zhu's need for a new heart to cure his stupidity). The judge agreed and went off to wherever he got his body parts in the netherworld, picked out the most beautiful head he could find and returned with it tucked under his arm.

Kneeling at Zhu's wife's bedside, Lu gave Zhu the new head to hold while he drew a steel blade from his boot. The judge cut through the woman's neck as she slept. Her head fell behind her pillow and the judge suggested Zhu get rid of it as he took the pretty replacement from his arms. To complete the transplant, he lined the head up to the neck and pressed it down to make it stick. When Zhu's wife woke, she felt a strange sensation around her neck. Fingering it while looking in the mirror, she was surprised to find a red seam and an unfamiliar face.[1]

Spare Parts tells the story of transplants from the sixteenth century onwards. The sixteenth century marks a time both when myths about transplantation were openly ridiculed and real-life transplants re-emerged in Italy. In his novel *Pantagruel*, the French writer and doctor François Rabelais lampooned mystical transplant stories with one of his own creation. He tells the story of Episthemon, who was found dead with his bloody head between his arms. The surgeon, Panurge, said 'weep not one drop more, for he being yet all hot, I will make him as sound as ever he was'. And, with that, he grabbed the bloody head and stuffed his codpiece into its mouth – giving the pseudo medical explanation 'that the air might not enter into it' – while he cleaned the neck with white wine, then lined up the head and sewed it on. Episthemon started to breathe again, 'opened his eyes, yawned, sneezed, and afterwards let out a great fart'.[2]

When skin grafting began in Renaissance Italy in the form

of nose jobs, it seemed to have lost the regal status it had enjoyed in ancient India. In Italy, skin grafting had evolved as a peasant's operation, linked culturally and technically to the farmer's procedure of plant grafting, and the few surgeons who performed it kept their techniques secret. An indiscreet renegade surgeon, popular with the masses, would soon change this and skin grafts would become more widely practised by the end of the sixteenth century, but to begin with the medical establishment had no concept of surgical transplantation. Even Andreas Vesalius, the most famous and well-respected anatomist of the time, thought replacement noses were crafted from muscles (which would have been impossible).

Only a few decades after the re-emergence of skin grafting, and after a great deal of experimentation, the English physician William Harvey came to the conclusion that the heart behaves like a pump, forcing the blood around the body in a circuit. It took only a few short decades more for doctors and scientists in England and France to use this idea to pioneer another kind of transplant: the blood transfusion. By accepting the theory of circulation, these early pioneers attempted to connect two bodies as if they were coupling machines. Thanks to some persistent, old-world medical ideas, these early experiments were informed by myths and legends and included transfusions between animals and humans. Though these were ultimately unsuccessful (at least by our standards), blood transfusions would – like skin grafts – eventually become essential to the development of organ transplantation by contributing to our understanding of the mechanisms that make bodies compatible or incompatible with one another. And it was in these early modern days of the seventeenth century that scientists started to form the first notion of blood types.

The idea that the body was constructed of 'parts' suggested that all kinds of compatibilities might exist, and in the eighteenth century this sparked the first market in body parts for transplantation. As consumer culture gathered momentum, dentists went out hunting for teeth, extracting them from corpses, buying them by the barrel from battlefields ('Waterloo Teeth'). They also cajoled them from poor children to transplant directly into the mouths of the rich. And by the nineteenth century, the physiological mechanism that supposedly made the tooth transplant work had reignited hopes of successful blood transfusions – between two humans this time. It was in these dark years of Regency London that transplantation first found a clear, recognizable purpose: from here on, transplants would (mostly) be carried out to save human lives.

Even when it finally became conceivable to transplant internal organs in the very first years of the twentieth century, there were more surprises. The technique surgeons use to stitch organs into bodies today was informed by the unacknowledged work of the seamstress and lacemaker Marie-Anne Leroudier. Later in the century Willem Kolff, a Dutch doctor and inventor, created an artificial kidney from a tangle of sausage skins, an enamel bath and parts scavenged from shot-down German aircraft. His later machines that bypassed the heart and lungs would also make it possible for people like Christiaan Barnard to at last transplant a human heart. Further technical advances enabled surgeons to transplant even more complex structures, such as faces and arms, and bioengineers and stem-cell scientists have successfully grown human heart tissue on the collagen scaffold of a spinach leaf.

While organ transplants are clearly a significant chapter in the story of transplantation, in this book I see them as part of a much longer history and wider cultural context. In the last seventy years or so, technology has enabled us to transplant organs, but transplants per se have been widespread for at least 500 years and are underpinned by 5,000 years of culture without which modern transplants like the one I witnessed at London's Royal Free Hospital would be inconceivable.

In widening the scope of the transplant narrative, I hope also to show that the story of transplantation is not merely one of technical progress leading to mastery but a primarily human journey. The story of transplants is about something closer to our hearts than pumps and valves; it's about how we understand our bodies, and about our relationships with one another and with ourselves. Raw information on these procedures is abundant – the doctors and scientists who worked on transplants didn't keep their thoughts to themselves, and the artists, playwrights and writers who described them didn't leave their brushes and pens idle. With such a rich set of sources as well as various academic reports, this isn't just a matter of the odd ghoulish curiosity, but a detailed history that amplifies the big questions we all ask about ourselves: when you think about what it actually *means* to move bits of body around, transplantation becomes a far bigger issue than accounts of impressive technology and highly talented medical professionals. Looked at this way, transplant surgery becomes nothing less than an intuitive meditation on our sense of personal identity, a perhaps unwitting fumble towards understanding what it means to be human, alive and an individual. It is with this very question of human and individual identity that the history begins in Renaissance Italy.

1. Skin (1550–1597)

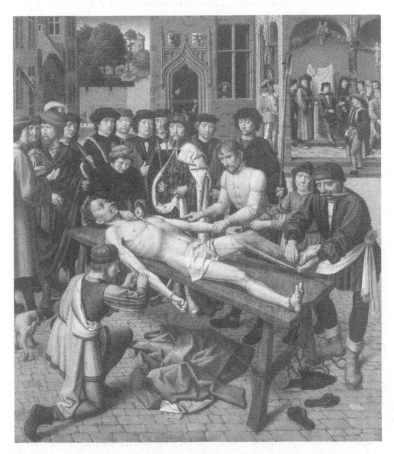

Figure 1 Gerard David: the flaying of Sisamnes from 'The Judgement of Cambyses', 1498, oil on wood.

The flaying of Sisamnes, a corrupt Persian judge, comprises one half of 'The Judgement of Cambyses', a 1498 diptych by Gerard David. Sisamnes is tied to a table, his modesty covered by a towel lest the sight of a penis should offend us as we witness four knife-wielding torturers peel the skin from his legs, arms and torso. His clenched teeth and veins popping in agony differentiate this still-living person from a body on an anatomist's table. The action is freeze-framed just moments before his identity and humanity are peeled away like the skin of a rabbit, leaving only impersonal flesh and bone. After the flaying, the king appointed the judge's son to replace his father at court. You can see him enthroned on the top right of the painting. The new judge's chair is a gift from the king, who, for reasons of poetry and deterrence, had it upholstered in Sisamnes's skin.

This image was painted around the time of the first modern skin grafts. It depicts a relationship between a person and their skin on the cusp of being dissolved, and gets its power from showing the fragility of the connection between our skins and ourselves.[1] It's hard to imagine ourselves without our skins. They distinguish us from meat, and such a prospect of extreme mutilation threatens to erase our very identities as humans. There are actually very few documented cases of flaying (though the Scythians were once famed for their skinning skills), but the first modern transplants were performed because the world was generally far more hostile to skin than it is now, and to noses in particular.

In the Renaissance (and earlier), losing a nose was a constant possibility. Some would have lost theirs in fights or duels. Many other noses would have been taken as punishment, an assault on a perpetrator's sense of self. Cutting off the nose – rhinotomy – occasionally makes a shocking appearance in the news today but was once a routine punishment with a long history in ancient India, and at various times in Europe and the Middle East. The Egyptian penal code punished adultery through mutilation of the nose.[2] In the mid-1160s BC, the Pharaoh Rameses III ordered the rhinotomy of his magistrates' noses. They had colluded with Queen Teya – his secondary queen who wanted her son to be pharaoh – to slit his throat while he sat in his royal harem playing board games.[3] The nose situation in Egypt, in fact, must have been particularly dire: *Harper's Dictionary of Classical Antiquities* cites a city of 'cut-off-noses' – Rhinokoloura – a settlement built on the edge of the desert, populated entirely by criminals who'd been mutilated under the Aethiopian dynasty.

If you look for them, you'll find people chopping off noses all over the place. In Rome it was permissible for a wronged man to cut off the nose of his cheating wife or her lover.[4] Pope Sixtus V tried to deter highway robbers from invading Rome and the surrounding countryside by threatening nasal mutilation.[5] Italian traveller and surgeon Niccolao Manucci similarly wrote about Mughal horsemen losing their noses when passing through the forests of Mysore. The forest inhabitants would run at them, spring up from behind and cut them off with a specially designed, half-moon-shaped blade.

We might also add syphilis – a virulent threat in sixteenth-century Europe – to the reasons someone might require a new nose. The disease was far more severe than the cases we see today. It started with sores around the genitals, moving on to ulcers, fever, blindness, abscesses and dementia. One of the most horrifying symptoms, though, was the rotting and collapse of the nose, leaving only a hole. As syphilis could be, but wasn't always, transmitted sexually, the so-called 'saddle nose' of a sufferer came to signify low moral standards, compounding the general shame of being nose-less. Losing a nose was so horrific that the sixteenth-century theologian Thomas Sanchez considered it grounds for the annulment of a marriage.[6]

Losing a nose removed the senses of taste and smell and impaired the voice, but the social isolation and rejection it brought would have been far worse. The only realistic solu-tion for many was a nose mask. These were hardly convincing replacements – some were just false noses dangling from spectacle frames and looked more like party masks – but seem to have had formed part of the nasal landscape (literally in the case of Egypt, since archaeologists have dug up mum-mies with false noses[7]). Even famous people wore them.

Tycho Brahe was one example. He was the last major astronomer to use only the naked eye, and in the final year of his life took on the much more famous Johannes Kepler as an assistant. But in his youth, he got into a mathematical dis-agreement at a Christmas party with another twenty-year-old Dane, Manderup Parsberg. Whatever their difference, it was severe enough for them to leave the party and walk off to a pitch-black graveyard, where, amongst the gravestones, they drew swords. Blind with indignation as well as the absence of light, they flailed around, frantically jabbing and slashing in each other's general direction. After a few seconds, Pars-berg's sword made contact, taking a good chunk out of the astronomer's nose.

The two men eventually made up and years later became great friends, and even family, when Parsberg's cousin mar-ried Brahe's brother.[8] In the meantime, though, Brahe was disfigured, and embarrassed at the idea of walking around with an ugly wound that would also be a constant reminder of his defeat. Consequently, he had a replacement nose created. A

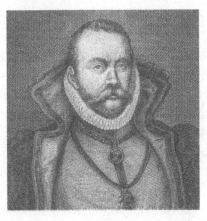

Figure 2 Tycho Brahe (line engraving by J. L. Appold after J. de Gheyn, 1586).

lowly material such as wax, his biographer claims, would have been beneath a man of his station, so he chose one of 'silver and gold', painted to match the shade of his skin. (This claim has since been debunked by Danish and Czech researchers, who in 2010 performed a chemical analysis on the artificial nose, which turned out to be brass.[9]) Portraits of Brahe show this splendid creation glued to his face, and it looks quite convincing. But, if one of his friends is to be believed, the nose would now and then work itself loose, so he took to carrying a little box filled with glue he could apply whenever it started to wobble.

The life of Emperor Justinian II in the late seventh century surely wins the prize for the story with the highest number of chopped-off noses and the most effective nose mask in history. It wasn't a prerequisite for a Byzantine ruler to be of royal birth, but it *was* important to be free from physical imperfection. A physically imperfect man, the Byzantines believed, could never become emperor. With this in mind, Justinian's father, Constantine IV, established his son as joint emperor and ordered the mutilation of his own brothers' noses. In due course, Justinian became emperor, seated in Constantinople. Later, Justinian was usurped by one of his own soldiers, Leontios, who mutilated Justinian's nose and tongue to secure his own position on the throne. Then Leontios was deposed by a naval officer calling himself Tiberius. Of course, Tiberius chopped off Leontios's nose.

Justinian II – so badly deformed he was known as Rhinokopimenos, the man with the cut-off nose – had in the meantime been plotting his comeback from exile. He returned to Constantinople, entering the city through a disused water conduit that ran under the walls. Once inside, he roused supporters and fought for and reclaimed the throne, overturning the idea that the imperial leader had to be free from physical deformity. According to the writings of Agnellus of Ravenna, he was wearing a replacement nose made of pure gold.[10]

For those who knew about it, though, there was another possibility to help undo the curse of noselessness: a skin graft – an operation last heard of in ancient Rome. We have records of two families practising their own secret techniques in Renaissance Italy. The Branca family were from Catania in Sicily and are remembered as the surgeons who 'rediscovered' the skin-graft operation and later improved it by taking skin from the forearm rather than the forehead. Around 1460 a member of the family taught the skin-graft procedure to a German physician, a Teutonic knight called Heinrich von Pfolspeundt. A leading surgeon of the age, Guy de Chauliac, dismissed the knight as 'curing all wounds with incantations, potions, oil, wool, and cabbage leaves'.[11] Pfolspeundt published a description of the operation in German, but it never received much attention, and he represents something of a dead end in the history of trans-plantation. The second family, the Vianeo family, lived in Tropea, a tiny fishing village in Calabria, also famous for its red onions. Like the Branca family, Pietro and Paolo Vianeo had a special technique to take the skin from a person's fore-arm and transplant it onto their face. They'd learned how to do this from their father, Bernardino, who had in turn been taught by his uncle Vincenzo.

Throughout the sixteenth century – and probably even earlier – a steady stream of wealthy and emasculated men would have wound their way to the family surgery, hands clasped over their noseless faces. Many of them would have been disfigured trying to protect their honour in fights or duels. Some might have been punished. Others would have come in shame, with the eroded 'saddle nose' of a syphilis sufferer. They might have tried a nose mask in the past but wanted a more natural-looking substitute. With their special procedures to replace a lost nose, the Branca and Vianeo families offered these men a much-valued restoration of dig-nity, a solution far more effective (but also a procedure far more daunting) than the alternative of a face mask.

The Human Tree

One day in 1549, the Vianeo brothers opened their door to find a bearded gentleman with a perfectly intact nose – a well-proportioned one sticking out above a full beard. The stranger clearly didn't need their services himself, but with his servant on one side and his horse on the other, he stood at the door's threshold and shared his story. He was from Bologna, and his relative had lost his nose fighting in

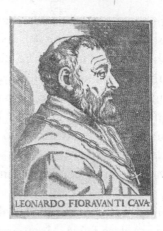

LEONARDO FIORAVANTI CAVA

Figure 3 Leonardo Fioravanti, 1582.

Lombardy. The man had heard the family could perform miracles in such cases and wanted to see them in action before recommending that his own flesh and blood submit to their knives. It sounded like a reasonable request, so the surgeons invited him into their surgery. What the brothers didn't know was that the man they'd just invited into their secret world was a fellow surgeon who wanted in on their special technique. Leonardo Fioravanti was his name, and he'd concocted this whole back-story knowing the family would never be open with another medical man.[12] It's thanks to this man's medical spy capers that, eventually, skin transplants found their way from the secretive Vianeo family to more mainstream surgeons who adopted a slightly modified version of the technique – a technique, incidentally, that was in use as late as the Second World War.

When the moment came, Fioravanti threw himself into his role, pretending to be shocked by the whole bloody affair. He made the appropriate displays of agitation, putting his hands to his face as any squeamish observer might. But peering through gaps in his splayed fingers, he made careful note of what he saw.

Wielding pincers, the brothers pinched some of the skin from the man's left arm and used a knife to slice it away from the muscle. They didn't separate the skin from the arm completely, though. It became a flap, attached at one end, the other drooping away from the body. Next, they passed a piece of linen under the flap, and medicated the skin until it toughened up. Once it was thick and strong enough, they moved their knives to the area where the nose should be, and cut around it, creating an open wound on the face. Working quickly now, they cut off the end of the arm flap to create a second open wound. So the wounds could heal together, and the patient's face and arm unite as one, the brothers bound arm to face, the open wounds touching one another. The surgeons instructed their patient not to move his arm until its skin had 'grown into the nose'. Once the body parts had fused, the surgeons cut the skin away from the arm and moulded it around 'a form of metal' until the new nose grew to the right dimensions. The result was convincing to Fioravanti, though he noticed the new nose was a little whiter than the rest of its owner's face.

It's not clear whether Fioravanti knew about the ancient Indian technique that used skin from the forehead instead of the forearm. He did, however, know that the same kind of operation had been practised for centuries on plants. The Chinese and Indians were grafting plants at least as far back as 2000 BC. And plant grafting was already commonplace in ancient Greece. In AD 70 the Roman agricultural writer Columella described the surgery: it required a tree with 'moist, juicy and strong bark', like a fig or an olive. A young and healthy branch was amputated from one tree, some of its bark removed and the same shape cut into the branch of a second, host, tree. If these two were bound together, the two open wounds touching, the trees would unite within twenty-one days. Following this technique (or one of three others Columella described in his book *On Agriculture*), would produce trees with more high-yield branches, and therefore more fruit. It was even possible to graft different species onto one another. Typically, these species would be closely related, for example apples and pears, but Pliny the Elder reported seeing a tree at Tivoli 'bearing every sort of fruit; walnuts on one branch, berries on another, on others grapes, pears, figs, pomegranates, and apples'.[13]

Reporting on his observations later, Fioravanti was explicit about this connection between the agricultural and surgical operations. The only real difference between the two procedures was the material – bark versus skin. The healing process was otherwise the same. When bark is wounded and brought together with bark, the two organisms fuse to become one. When skin is cut and brought together with skin, the same thing happens. For the Vianeo brothers, Fioravanti or anyone else who wanted to perform a skin graft, this healing mechanism was an opportunity to use the skin as a material to help shape and sculpt the human form. A crafty surgeon could even apply these principles to form an entirely new appendage. Cultivating humans was so close to cultivating the land, in fact, that Fioravanti described this kind of transplant surgery as the 'agriculture of the body' and the 'farming of men'.

As a surgical technique drawing on sophisticated agricultural procedures, the skin graft was ingenious. But it was also intuitive. Transplanting skin was part of a surprisingly universal inclination to learn more about ourselves by looking to plants and trees. In his twelve-volume masterpiece of

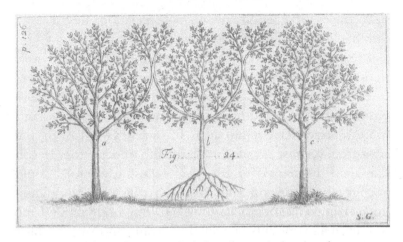

Figure 4 An eighteenth-century depiction of an agricultural graft, 1772.

early twentieth-century anthropology, *The Golden Bough*, the Scottish anthropologist Sir James George Frazer noticed this wider tendency. Having amassed thousands of stories and anthropological studies, Frazer marshalled them into an overarching narrative of human progress. 'Primitive' cultures, he concluded, engineered their societies around a belief in magic, but eventually realized magic didn't work, and started to invent and appeal to gods of one kind or another instead. When they finally realized this didn't work either, they alighted at the pinnacle of humanity – a society based on and guided by science. The dusty volumes have a whiff of Indiana Jones about them, with index entries like 'ass in rainmaking ceremony', 'mock battle at festival of new fruits', 'walrus, taboos concerning'. And they're what you might expect of an industrious old-school anthropologist who referred to people as 'savages' – the scale of vision admirable, but the argument simplistic and warped. Though his conclusions were based on a flawed premise, it's nevertheless staggering how many civilizations he surveyed that had a deep cultural affinity with trees.

From Australia to Zanzibar and throughout all time, people have taken their ties with trees seriously. We've set trees on fire when people die, secreted dead bodies in trees, embraced them in the hope of getting pregnant, even hammered extracted teeth into them. In ancient Germany the life of a tree was just as valuable as the life of a person. If you damaged the bark of a tree your fellow townsfolk would avenge it by cutting out your navel and nailing it to the injured limb. They would then have driven your body around the tree until all your guts entwined its trunk, and you wouldn't live to harm another. That was the idea – 'a life for a life', your pulled innards replacing the dead bark with a living substitute. Fundamental and constant, human–tree bonds are everywhere. Human beings have used trees in rituals, as avatars, for medicine. An Indian tribe even married mango trees off to tamarind and jasmine trees to sanctify their crops.[14]

When trees age, their bark ages much like human skin – sagging, folding, wrinkling, blemishing. Making this observation in the first century AD, the Roman naturalist Pliny the Elder wrote about how trees have the equivalents of 'skin, flesh, sinews, veins, bones, and marrow', and a juice 'which must be looked upon as their blood'.[15] Four hundred or so years earlier, Aristotle brought plants and animals closer together by directly comparing a seed to an egg, referring to a plant's roots as its 'mouth'. So similar were plants and animals in his eyes, in fact, that he referred to a plant as a 'rooted animal'.[16]

In their theories of digestion, some ancient philosophers like Aristotle saw a *continuum* between plants and humans as the former metamorphosed into the latter. Galen of Pergamon was the most influential doctor of all time – a Greek physician to the gladiators who lived, thought and wrote between the years 129 and roughly 210. As we'll see, his works would sit on the shelves of almost every doctor from the third to the eighteenth century. When he described the process of digestion, he painted a picture of a real-life meta-morphosis of plant into human. When we eat, Galen wrote, the top part of the stomach transforms into the shape of a hand. It reaches out to grab food from the gullet and draws it back into itself. This is the start of the transformation of food into flesh. Once the stomach-hand has grabbed the food, it's sorted into nutritious and non-nutritious parts. The non-nutritious part floats off towards the spleen and becomes black bile. The nourishing part ends up being concocted into chyle, then fermented into a fluid and invested with a primal 'vegetative spirit'. This spirit – the life force common to every living thing – rushes through the body's veins as blood to heal any wounds we might have, to help us grow and to keep us alive. A human would eat plants (and animals, who themselves ate plants) and the body would use this material to grow, nourish and replace bits a hostile world had nicked, grazed or lopped off.[17]

Further entangling plants and people, Aristotle even lumped sexual reproduction into the category of digestion. Semen and menstrual blood, he thought, were both ultimately created out of digested food. And these two substances would together produce an entirely new body. These plant-derived raw materials remained visible in the body throughout life. You could see the remnants of semen in the hard, white and vital parts like bone and organs, while menstrual blood supposedly made up the squishy bits in between. Injuries to parts derived from sperm were (mostly) permanent, whereas sanguinary parts could regenerate, a so-called 'nutritive

soul' – also from plants, and very similar to Galen's 'vegetative soul' – literally helping to fill in any gaps.[18]

Although we don't tend to interpret digestion in quite
those terms any more, many centuries later we're still discovering the extent of the correspondences between people and
plants. Trees, it turns out, form networks with one another,
connecting and communicating in their own language of
smell, sound and electrical signals. They also sweat, form
memories and in some ways can even be considered individuals. And while they don't exactly have brains, trees learn
and store information in their roots. As we deepen our
understanding about the extent of our physiological kinship
with trees, modern science seems to echo the timeless and
intuitive observations shared by Aristotle, Pliny the Elder
and the tribes in Frazer's books.[19] Early transplant surgeons
like Fioravanti, too, observed human bodies to be behaving
so much like plants they could explain the process of healing. And activities that draw on that process, like grafting,
could be directly transposed from the plant kingdom to the
animal kingdom.

With the phrases 'agriculture of the body' and 'farming of
men', Fioravanti not only evoked an intuitive, universal, timeless kinship between trees and people, but also meant to pay
tribute to actual farmers and to attribute skin-graft surgery
to ordinary, everyday people. A year after his fishing trip to
the Vianeo surgery, we find Fioravanti pottering around the
east coast of Tunisia, near the town of Mahdia, where he got
the chance to try out skin grafting for himself. It was 1550
and a conflict was raging between the Spanish and the Otto-
mans. Fioravanti's companion, Andres Gutiero, was Spanish,
and when they passed a group of (presumably Ottoman)
soldiers, one decided to pick a fight. Lashing out with his

blade, the soldier sliced into Gutiero's face. His nose dropped into the dirt, rolled in some sand and came to rest on the ground in front of him. Blood welled from the gap where the nose used to be.

Luckily, Fioravanti wasn't far away, and he sensed a chance to try out some of his new-found skills. He walked over to pick up the nose, turned it around in his hands, inspected the severed object and came up with an ingenious idea. 'I pissed on it,' he confided in a book thirty-two years later. Having washed away the sand, he stuck the urine-soaked nose back onto his friend's face and applied stitches and balsam before bandaging it up. Even Fioravanti didn't have much faith in this field surgery and was surprised when he untied the bandage to see the nose was attached again. If readers didn't believe him, he wrote – and there was a good chance they wouldn't – they could ask Gutiero, who was alive and well.[20]

He was right. It *is* hard to believe. It's even harder to believe when we understand how practised a liar Fioravanti was. He was the kind of man to boast about visiting a hospital of incurables and curing everyone there. He claimed to have done just this, in fact, on a visit to Palermo.[21] The Sicilians also learned of his genius, he tells us, because when he visited Sicily to learn about distillation, he managed to cure leprosy, scrofula and syphilis on the side. Elsewhere on his travels he discovered the antiseptic qualities of saltwater, aquavit and urine (which I presume is why he decided to piss on Gutiero's nose). In one case while performing surgery on a patient's spleen, he requested his assistants and spectators to unfasten their trousers and relieve themselves in the patient's open abdomen (the patient survived).[22] But just as the Vianeo brothers swallowed his story about being a gentleman from Bologna, his public seemed to accept the magnificent claims he made for himself. Wherever he went, the people assumed he must be bringing secrets from a distant land, and would gather around him, he wrote, 'as to an oracle'.[23]

It's also possible that 'the people' didn't mind a bit of dishonesty because he went to great lengths to identify with them. He verified their unlettered experiences, took the trouble to learn their homespun medical wisdom and even insisted on its superiority over things written in books. Fioravanti would drag his horse far and wide, over land and sea, deliberately seeking out distillers, shepherds, countrywomen, peasants, soldiers – anyone who might have something to teach him. And he'd sit down and listen to them. In the Sicilian town of Messina, he met an old man who told him that he only ever took one medicine, soldanella, once per year, in spring. And every time he did so, he said, 'it makes me vomit thoroughly and leaves my stomach so clean that for a year I cannot fall ill'. He'd reached the age of 104, all by observing this 'natural way' of healing.[24]

Fioravanti, reflecting on the practices of these rural folk, concluded that they learned their medicine from 'the first physicians' – animals. The old man was copying what dogs did when they became ill. When a dog feels sick, it 'goes to the forest and finds there a certain sort of herb, which', Fioravanti wrote, 'immediately makes it vomit and evacuate from behind'.[25] Dogs know when they're diseased and intuit how to bring themselves back to health. Fioravanti let encounters like the one with the vomiting old man influence the medicines he concocted and sold as far as Elizabethan London. So that his patients could also purge their bodies and live a long life, Fioravanti created and marketed his own drugs to induce vomiting or diarrhoea, giving them theatrical names like Angelic Electuary, Leonardo's Grand Liquor and

Fragrant Goddess.[26] With Arcadian origins, the skin graft took its place far away from the echoing halls of theory-bound universities, literally amongst the trees and those who dwelled closest to them.

With probably a few exceptions (like the deceived Vianeo family), the people seemed to admire him back. His writings validated some of the discontent ordinary folk felt, believing themselves powerless. Ruled as they were by so-called elites studying and living apart from the real world, they could easily believe Fioravanti when he told them an academic doctor's impenetrable technical language was all part of his desire for exclusivity.[27] Fioravanti preferred to base his own medical system on the collective, intuitive wisdom of centuries – a live tradition with no written component – as opposed to a raft of dead, book-learned knowledge. He believed 'more in a little experience', he wrote, 'than in all the theories of the world taken together'.[28]

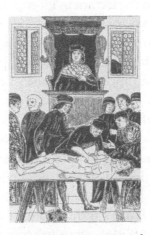

Figure 5 A dissection in progress: the anatomy professor at his lectern, 1493.

It's easy to sympathize with Fioravanti and the sceptical Renaissance public when we take a look at some of this 'conventional' medicine. At least Fioravanti trusted what he saw. What most physicians in the Renaissance (and earlier) knew of the world around them, and what they thought about it, mattered little. Anatomy demonstrations, for instance, involved an instructor, or lector, sitting in his chair reading aloud from an ancient medical text. On a table in front of him would be an executed criminal, and a surgeon or barber would open up the body as directed. Another assistant – an ostensor – would point a wand at the parts being discussed. It was really an anatomy demonstration in name only, the performance's main function being to repeat what was in the textbook. If what the audience saw was different from what the book described, they'd blame the inconsistency on bad translation, or even the body itself for being an anomaly.

Anatomy demonstrations like this had used the same format for over two hundred years. The anatomical textbook most likely to be on the lectern in Fioravanti's time – Mondino de Luzzi's *Anathomia Corporis Humani* – was the first book entirely devoted to anatomy, but had been written in 1316.[29] This book would have been the most important part of this entire exercise, even in the mid-1500s, since it parroted the theories of Galen.

Galen adapted the ideas of philosophers like Aristotle and developed them along with elements of other ancient thinkers such as Plato and Hippocrates to create a system touching upon and connecting all aspects of medicine. By the 800s, his body of work had spread to the Islamic world, starting with Hunayn ibn Ishaq's translations of his original Greek into Arabic. Once his ideas were an active part of the Islamic medical tradition, scholars debated and challenged them, modifying them according to their conclusions. By the eleventh century, Western scholars had got hold of the Arabic translations and made a Latin version. Unlike their Islamic counterparts, Western practitioners were closed to experimentation at the time, preferring to trust in the wisdom as it was written. So, these versions – Latin translations of Arabic translations of Greek – became established and unquestionable texts, deferred to not only in the anatomy demonstrations but also in all areas of medicine.

Although doctors through the ages invariably trusted Galen's writings over what they saw themselves, Galen himself, at least in part, based his theories on the observations he made cutting up bodies. But there was a problem here too. Dissecting humans was forbidden in imperial Rome. Galen had probably never even seen inside a human body, save for the glimpses he had when his gladiator patients stumbled or were carried from dusty arenas with their insides spilling out. All his anatomical descriptions were based on animals. The liver – the most important part in his anatomy because it created blood – he described as having five lobes, when in humans it really only has two. The septum of the heart (the wall that separates the right from the left chamber) was supposedly permeable. He'd argued that a 'vital principle' found in the air could mix with the blood by making its way through this septum. But there are no holes, so no way through for the blood. And the *rete mirabile*, the nervous structure at the base of the brain, translated as the 'wonderful net', exists in sheep, but no one has ever found one in a human.[30]

Western anatomy and medicine had, for hundreds of years, been effectively based on one man's anatomical romp through the animal kingdom. And his findings had been repeated, its truth insisted upon ad infinitum. The situation wasn't helped by the early Christian Church agreeing with and adopting some of Galen's ideas, which meant they also became a matter of faith and to challenge them could even be construed as questioning the Church. So, the doctors Fioravanti railed against really were arguing over inconsequential minutiae, over ancient interpretations of translations of translations of documents based on dissections of animals.

And all this influenced the everyday doctoring the sick were supposed to submit to and pay a fortune for the privilege of receiving. For everyday medical treatment, Galen popularized the theory of the four humours. These were blood, yellow bile, phlegm and black bile – four fluids that supposedly sloshed around our bodies in different concentrations depending on all sorts of factors. These included what you ate, your mood, your personality and even the motions of the stars. Accordingly, onto the four humours were mapped four classical temperaments – sanguine, choleric, phlegmatic and melancholic. Someone with a preponderance of blood was sanguine, for instance, and someone filled with black bile would be melancholic (from *melan* 'black' + *kholē* 'bile'). The humours were also linked to the four seasons, spring, summer, autumn, and winter. And the qualities of wetness, dryness, hotness and coldness were layered on top of these. By associating humours with seasons, temperaments and qualities, a physician would be able to read your 'complexion', which would help them diagnose the nature of your disease and how it related to your particular body. If a physician considered your humours to be balanced (they rarely did), you were healthy. If not, you were to some degree diseased and needed actively to restore equilibrium.

Everything – from what you ate to how you behaved – influenced your humoral balance. The ideal, then, was to maintain this balance by controlling your diet and exercise. Fresh barley, for example, 'is full of . . . moisture, absorbed from the soil which is filled with dampness and wind'. You could use these wet qualities to combat 'dry' diseases like pleurisy and inflammations of the lungs by 'moistening' them. Poppy seed, on the other hand, 'possesses a cooling power', is 'difficult to digest' but 'helps those who are subject to thin catarrh from the head'. If you wanted to, you could also confuse your body by eating foods together that counteract one another – like boiling cabbage and lentils in one pot, and seasoning the dish with olive oil, fish sauce and pepper. The liquid ingredients would pass through the bowels at the same time as the solids but would have opposite effects. This confusion wouldn't harm you, particularly, but your bowels would get mixed signals, to both open and close at the same time, which would cause you to fart. If controlling your health through diet failed or wasn't enough – and it was never *really* enough – a doctor could craft and sell a medicine especially for you, which would change your overall humoral mixture.[31]

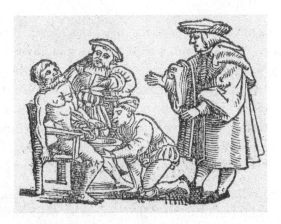

Figure 6 Bloodletting, sixteenth century.

By far the most common way to balance a patient's humours was to bleed them. Blood was associated with the essence of a person, their soul, and with life itself, but it was also one of the four humours, which made it also a symptom and, confusingly, even a cause of illness. Haemorrhoids, nosebleeds and menstruation were all considered signs of too much blood, since in these cases the body tried to get rid of it naturally. All the other humours ultimately ended up in the blood, too, though, so by removing blood you could also remove a general surplus of all humours (known as a plethora). You could only see the other humours when they became isolated during sickness, when black bile, yellow bile and phlegm left the body in excrement, vomit and mucus. A physician might chuck an emetic or laxative into your treatment plan to encourage you to expunge some of these for good measure. But for most complaints, large and small, you'd be bled back to equilibrium.

When one medieval medical handbook gave the rundown on the benefits of bloodletting, it looked like a miracle cure, claiming that it:

> clears the mind, strengthens the memory, cleanses the stomach, dries up the brain, warms the marrow, sharpens the hearing, stops tears, encourages discrimination, develops the senses, promotes digestion, produces a musical voice, dispels torpor, drives away anxiety, feeds the blood, rids it of poisonous matter, and brings long life. It eliminates rheumatic ailments, gets rid of persistent diseases, cures pain, fevers and various sicknesses and makes the urine clean and clear.[32]

Since bloodletting could treat anything from an upset stomach to discoloured urine, the dirty, everyday work of opening blood vessels was left to barbers. Barbers and surgeons were, in fact, coalesced in their own, low-status guild of barber-surgeons, and could relieve you of your blood and your beard on the same visit. The medical historian's favourite factoid is that bloodletting is the origin of the red-and-white-striped barber's pole we still see outside barber shops. The red and white symbolize the blood and the bandages wrapped around the pole a customer would cling to while being bled. Surgeons' hands-on approach distinguished them from the loftier physicians, whose university training demanded their noses be perpetually in books, and mostly Galen's books.

It's significant that Fioravanti found the secret of skin grafting in a little fishing village on the northern coast of Calabria. Learned physicians, detached from the world, would never have looked there. According to Fioravanti, a doctor's reluctance to listen to those closest to nature was due to their values being corrupted by arguing, reading and dissecting the finer points of completely irrelevant theories.[33] Their bloodlessness and bookishness were no substitute for the farmer's common sense and practical experience.[34] Not only were the physicians obsessing over books when they should have been paying attention to their patients' bodies, Fioravanti believed doctors also used their mastery of letters to show off. Jockeying for position, they tried their best to distinguish themselves as much as possible from the ignorant masses – the masses Fioravanti admired so much because they at least had common sense and were willing to trust their intuition.

With an attitude like his, it's hardly surprising Fioravanti had a terrible relationship with most university-trained physicians. The medical authorities got so fed up with him they accused him of quackery, and in 1573 Fioravanti found himself in prison in Milan for 'not medicating in the canonical way'. Before that, he'd been in Venice since 1558, where the

College of Physicians took exception to his methods, accusing him of fraud and endangering lives. This after spending the period 1555 to 1558 in Rome, from where he was chased away for similar transgressions.[35]

Fioravanti's behaviour made it hard for him to avoid gaining a reputation as a quack, but he actually *did* have a degree from Bologna University – the only university in the world, at the time, that would insist surgeons also had medical training. This might not seem particularly strange to us, but in the sixteenth century surgeons and doctors occupied very different parts of society from today. It was considered so beneath a doctor's dignity to dirty his hands with scalpels and drills, in fact, that in the fourteenth century the Faculty of Medicine in Paris actively *forbade* their graduates to perform surgery.[36]

Even considering Bologna's unique approach to surgical training, though, Fioravanti's views were extreme. Throughout his life, he repeated again and again that a surgeon's job was to 'help nature' and preached that doctors could learn more from people than they could from books. His admiration for nature and for the people who lived amongst it set him apart from pretty much everyone else in his profession. And the skin graft he discovered in a little fishing village was a prime example of the superiority of simple yet sophisticated rustic knowledge over the long-winded, convoluted, theory-laden medicine of academia that was completely divorced from reality.

Transplantation Makes It into a Divided Medical World

While Fioravanti was sniffing out the medicine of the people, a great shift was taking place in the world of conventional, university medicine he hated so much. In many ways, it was a shift towards his way of thinking. It started with two Galen fanatics – John Keys and Andreas Vesalius.[37] John Keys was one of England's foremost physicians. He'd served several members of the royal family, including the boy king Edward VI and Queen Mary. He served Elizabeth I for a while, too, but he was Catholic, and Catholics were out of favour during Elizabeth's reign. In the early 1540s Keys Latinized his name to Caius, which has the same pronunciation. You might recognize it from Cambridge University's Gonville and Caius College – he refounded his alma mater in 1557 and they adopted his name. But back in the 1540s he was an ultra-conservative physician, obsessed with Galen – the physician whose anatomical observations of animals dominated the European medical establishment.

Caius was determined to uphold Galen's legitimacy, not that there were many people questioning it at the time. There were, of course, the likes of Fioravanti, but his ideas were so subversive that no one in these rarefied circles could take him seriously. Like many others, if Caius heard any criticism levelled against Galen, he would explain it as resulting from a translation error. Others wanted to return to Greek sources around the same time for a similar reason. But Caius went one step further. He actually went to Padua in search of Galen's originals.

There he shared a room with Andreas Vesalius, a conservative Flemish anatomist. Vesalius, who was afflicted by dwarfism, had trained at the medical school in Paris, which had inculcated in him a regard for Galen to rival Caius's own. The Holy Roman Empire had sent an army to northern France, however, and, fearing his Belgian origins would be held against him if he stayed there, he fled to Leuven, close to his home city, Brussels, where he continued his studies. He then escaped this relative backwater to join the world-renowned medical school at Padua. Just days after passing his entrance exams he was appointed demonstrator and lecturer in surgery and anatomy. Similarly gifted and with the same intentions, he and Caius got on well and ended up working together, translating Galen by the light of a shared candle.

But there was a key difference between the two friends. For Caius, Galen's words were close to divine. He once said Galen was 'a man so great that the world of medicine has had none such since his death nor will have again'. Vesalius, on the other hand, had no interest in slavishly reproducing what he might deem faulty. Still, Vesalius's admiration for Galen seems to have held, at least at first. But when checking the original text against that of one of his teachers, Vesalius started to notice Galen's lack of experience with human bodies. Taking his own knife to corpses, he found a two-lobed liver, no evidence of a permeable septum between the heart's left and right chambers, and the *rete mirabile* was entirely absent. As his knife plunged into one cadaver after another, it started to puncture his confidence in his hero. And he wrote about what he saw.

His book *On the Fabric of the Human Body* was something of a tipping point because it presented the anatomist's own observations, which encouraged his fellow anatomists to question what they, too, were being told. Published in 1543, the *Fabrica* was an earth-shattering book, becoming one of the reasons we traditionally consider that year to be the start of the Scientific Revolution. The same year, Copernicus's *De revolutionibus orbium coelestium* ('On the Revolutions of the Heavenly Spheres') had much the same effect on the study

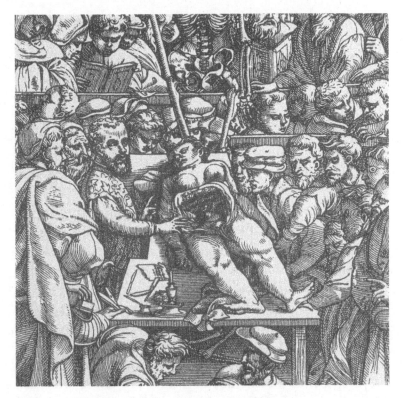

Figure 7 Andreas Vesalius dissecting a female cadaver, 1555.

of the stars. The Renaissance world put humankind at the centre of the universe, literally in the case of astronomy, but here were two books published in the same year suggesting that was all nonsense.

To many, Vesalius was an iconoclast, but he opened his book by arguing for the revival of anatomy teaching based on ancient models, and with no alternative explanations for most things he actually relied on Galen's work quite heavily. In several ways he was more loyal to Galen than Caius. The ancient Greek himself had criticized the followers of a rival anatomist, Erasistratus – who was, incidentally, the first person to compare a heart to a water pump – for 'revering their leader' as a 'God',[38] supposing 'everything he says is true'. Galen seems to have valued using one's own judgement and experience, and Vesalius would surely have known and drawn confidence from this. The *Fabrica* was a challenge aimed not primarily at him, but at those who blindly accepted his teachings without allowing for the possibility of his being human like the rest of us. The real targets were people like Caius, who didn't recognize any possibility of error.

The medical world was divided as two camps emerged. The first, represented by Caius, were backward-looking. As Caius's career advanced, he gained power – by 1555 he was in London, the president of the Royal College of Physicians – but he never truly moved on. He was so engrossed by tradition that he invented his own, including funeral rites for dead college fellows and installing the three ceremonial gates at Gonville and Caius. And his fanaticism for Galen never abated. In December 1559 Caius oversaw the trial of John Geynes, a little-known doctor from Newhaven, who said Galen 'had erred'. Galen had been dead for 1,349 years, and Vesalius's book had been published well over a decade earlier, but the official line at the Royal College of Physicians with Caius at its head was still that Galen could do no wrong. After almost a year of resistance, Geynes was hectored into making a public retraction. He signed a document acknowledging that Galen hadn't made any mistakes after all. The chastened doctor was made an example of for the benefit of anyone arrogant enough to question the unquestionable authority of Galen, and, by extension, a professional body of physicians sanctioned by royalty.

The second, more progressive camp belonged to Vesalius

and his followers, and it started to flourish alongside the unbelievably persistent Galenic system. Vesalius's *Fabrica* was a breakthrough in 1543, and the anatomist's faith in what his scalpel had discovered opened up an intellectual space in which physicians of the future could question what they read. This revolutionized university medicine. As anatomist after anatomist came around to Vesalius's way of thinking, they started to identify more of Galen's errors and confidence grew in this new concept of a medicine based on observation, on evidence, on science. Eventually, as it became fashionable to question ancient authority in all parts of life, to become an opponent of Vesalius was considered retrogressive. And to be a Galenist was to be an opponent of Vesalius, like Caius – who died in 1573, protector of a dying world.

Although Vesalius's camp eventually won out – no doctor would refer to Galen nowadays – the day-to-day reality for physicians and surgeons didn't change overnight. It wouldn't, in fact, change on a large scale for quite some time, until at least the eighteenth century. Some parts – such as bloodletting – lingered into the nineteenth century and, in places, even the early twentieth.[39] We still use Galen's two-fingers-on-the-wrist method of checking for a pulse, and some older people might remember a time in the 1950s when you could have walked into a pharmacy and seen a range of syrups, extracts and tinctures. These were called 'galenicals' and the pharmacist would mix them for you according to what your body and its disease demanded.

At the core of this controversy was the question of authority versus experience: whether you should listen to your elders or see for yourself. You might expect a figure like Fioravanti to come down firmly on the 'experience' side in this debate

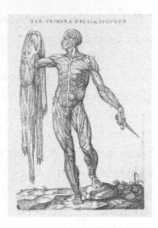

Figure 8 Male *écorché*, 1556.

and back Vesalius, but he effectively formed a camp of his own. He detested *all* modern medicine, by which he meant anything from the last two millennia or so. He reserved a special ire, as it happens, for Vesalius and spat out insults directed at his followers. One, Realdo Colombo – the man who coined the word 'placenta', which is Latin for a type of flat cake – he called a 'dogfish'. As far as Fioravanti was concerned, the entire debate was one of those university-bound discussions that had no meaning in the real world. 'Among all of us doctors,' he wrote, 'we don't argue over anything except those things which the human mind cannot grasp.'[40]

Vesalius also represented a class of medical practitioner that had little respect for the skin, which was merely something for his scalpel to pierce on its way to the more important internal organs. This disregard for skin was expressed by the Italian Renaissance surgeon Alessandro Benedetti, who likened it to the crust on polenta. This was actually a version of an idea repeated for centuries emanating from Aristotle, who came up with an even less beautiful image – he said that skin was 'like the scum upon boiled substances'.[41] Illustrated anatomy books from the Renaissance (and even later) mirror this disrespect. Open one up and you'll probably see images of human figures with their skin removed. This kind of illustration is called *écorché*, and the figures are often drawn carrying their own skins as if they don't quite know what to do with them.[42] It wouldn't have escaped Fioravanti's attention that Vesalius had actually written about the skin graft, too, but – typical university man – had clearly never seen one. And it seems Vesalius didn't even think the skin graft was actually a skin graft – he thought new noses were fashioned out of a muscle from the forearm. It was a misunderstanding that would have played into Fioravanti's claim that all university medicine was out of touch and useless.[43]

Fioravanti's special hatred for anatomists was also partly due to their further lowering the status of surgeons. This wasn't all Vesalius's fault – in sixteenth-century Italy, surgery was beginning to lose its association with the barbers that Fioravanti identified with. The medical authorities had started to issue decrees to get control over licensing surgeons, eventually making surgery a proper university subject, though it would take many decades for surgeons to find the same social status as physicians. Fioravanti saw this trend not as an elevation of his profession, but as the physicians trying to assume full control over medical matters, sending medicine, as he put it, 'straight to the bordello'.[44] Vesalius was just part of this general historical shift, though a very influential one. He'd effectively banished surgeons from the anatomist's theatre altogether, relegating them to sharpening blades for their new anatomist masters. At least in the old system surgeons had something worthwhile to do, albeit something they were instructed to do from on high. For Fioravanti, this was an assault on the dignity of the surgeon and further evidence that these bookish people were willingly ignoring the only legitimate source of knowledge – nature and those who lived closest to it.[45] And he resisted. 'If you want to know anatomy,' he said, 'it would be better to study agriculture.'[46]

Transplant surgery, based as it was on practical experience and drawn from humble farmers, simply had no place in the world of university medicine. That is, at least until Fioravanti put it there himself. In the 1560s Fioravanti met the Bolognese professor of surgery Giulio Cesare Aranzio. Aranzio wrote his own anatomical books, taking the Vesalian approach, relying on his own research and that of his contemporaries (though he also quoted Galen alongside them). Fioravanti knew of Aranzio by reputation, and claimed he was so skilful he 'almost brings the dead back to life when he lays hands on them'.[47] The two men became friends. At some point in their friendship, Fioravanti passed on the Vianeo brothers' secret, and Aranzio started to sculpt his own noses in Bologna. In the 1570s Aranzio became more important in the university, taking the first chair in anatomy – a post he created by separating 'surgery' and 'anatomy' into different professorships. In 1588 Fioravanti died. With his friend out of the way, Aranzio could conveniently ignore where he got the idea and allow people to believe he was 'the first restorer of noses and ears'.[48] But he died, too, a year later in 1589.

Thankfully, he taught the technique to one of *his* students, Gaspare Tagliacozzi, who, upon Aranzio's death, took over from his former teacher as Chair of Anatomy. Vesalius's empirical approach had, by this time, already been embraced by the medical school at Bologna and Tagliacozzi himself benefited from such an education. One of his teachers,

Girolamo Cardano, an early pioneer of clinical psychiatry, wrote the first clinical description of typhus fever by following his own observations. Another, Ulisse Aldrovandi, is still famous today as a natural philosopher, the man who in 1603 coined the word 'geology'. Aldrovandi was a prodigious collector of animals, plants, minerals and fossils. He tried to theorize a new science based on observation, collection, description and classification of all natural objects – about as far away from blindly following a book as it's possible to get.[49] He's now considered one of the first natural scientists and was in fact the first professor of natural sciences at Bologna. Tagliacozzi continued in this Vesalian direction, using his position as professor to conduct his own anatomical dissections.[50]

By this point he'd already started to codify the skin grafting method. And he eventually published it in 1597 as *De Curtorum Chirurgia per Insitionem* ('On the Surgery of Mutilation by Grafting'). Tagliacozzi's description is similar to Fioravanti's, only slightly modified. But his book is much better known, and arguably had a far greater impact, and with its intricate woodcuts the operation was laid bare for any surgeon to copy, a secret no more. The drawings showed the results surgeons should aim for and patients could expect, and covered not only replacing lost noses, but also fixing mutilated lips and ears. They illustrated the range of positions a patient would have to adopt, bound in various braces with their arm looking like it was doing an impression of an elephant's trunk. Really, though, it was more like the arm doing an impression of a tree trunk: at the end of the first part of Tagliacozzi's book, he drew the same comparison as Fioravanti, that surgery – and most especially skin grafting – is like the cultivation of trees.

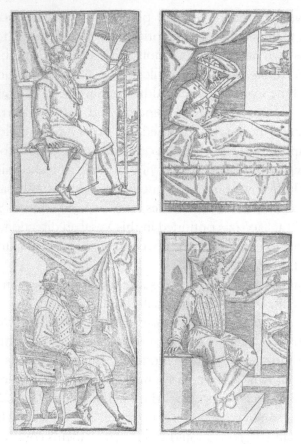

Figures 9–12 Gaspare Tagliacozzi's skin graft, images from *De Curtorum Chirurgia per Insitionem.*

Though he didn't recommend it, Tagliacozzi also wrote about how it would be technically possible to craft someone's new nose from the skin of their slave or servant, just as the branch of a pear tree could be grafted onto an apple tree. But the surgeon shunned the idea for a couple of reasons. First, the problem with using a second person as a donor: you wouldn't want to be attached, motionless, to anyone else for weeks on end while your separate bodies grew flesh bridges between themselves. And second, the 'force' and 'power' of 'individuality'. Though this latter objection to using a donor could have been a philosophical statement, it's possible that the force and power of individuality refers to the way bodies tend to reject parts transplanted from one to another.[51] Whether Tagliacozzi meant this or not, this fundamental incompatibility between two bodies would have been the most likely physiological reason a graft between two people wouldn't have taken. And, though there was no such concept in the sixteenth century, 'rejection' would effectively be an insurmountable clinical problem for transplant surgeons right up until the 1980s.

When Fioravanti stole the Vianco family's secret skin-grafting technique, it was deeply embedded in a rustic tradition, an operation of the people. As far as Fioravanti was concerned, it also exhibited the inevitable superiority of the common folk over the pretentious, corrupt, university-trained doctor. When Tagliacozzi wrote up the technique at the end of the sixteenth century, it was now intended for a new audience of scholars and conventionally trained doctors and surgeons. Tagliacozzi *did* recognize the agricultural origins of skin grafting, as Fioravanti had before him, but he'd have to deal with a new set of concerns his more renegade predecessor would have just dismissed: was crafting a new nose tantamount to playing God?

Earlier in the century, Italian gardeners, architects and sculptors faced the same question, and they used their art to evoke the monstrous consequences one might expect from altering natural forms. They built great statues, fountains and even water-controlled pipe organs that acknowledged the potential implications of interfering with Creation. The fountains controlled the elements, sending jets of water high into the air; the water organs metamorphosed water into sound; the statues were of impossible or terrifying beings. An anonymous British visitor to the gardens of Tivoli's Villa d'Este in 1610 described one such sculpted dragon fountain as 'belching water being of so black a colour, that it resembleth an ugly smoke, fearful to behold'.[52] These creations reflected their makers' preoccupation with just what it was they were making, which seemed to fall outside the categories of 'natural' and 'artificial'.

When the historian Jacopo Bonfadio visited the gardens on the shores of Lake Garda in 1541, he couldn't find words to describe a landscape that seemed neither fully natural nor fully artificial. The scholar Bartolomeo Taegio faced the same quandary in 1559 when he wrote *La Villa*, a tract on country life. The Roman statesman Cicero had described the 'first nature' of the wilderness, and 'second nature' of cultivated land like farms, orchards and dammed rivers,[53] but formal gardens were different. Gardeners used natural materials, but they weren't undisturbed nature *or* cultivated land, so you couldn't really call them examples of first or second nature. Both Bonfadio and Taegio – independently, it seems – opted to describe the garden as 'third nature'.[54] This new category recognized that the materials were natural, but they'd been guided by art, by human hands.[55] 'Natural artifice' and 'artificial nature' were two other attempts at labelling the peculiarity of a garden.[56] For the garden, nature provided the raw materials – terrain, trees, plants, flowers, stones, water – and a palette of colours, forms, textures and scents. Then artists cut, shaped and organized them.[57] If the writer Luke Morgan is to be believed, monsters like the dragons carved into water-spurting fountains are difficult to categorize along classical lines. This makes them examples of imperfect creatures or abominations, and putting them into Renaissance gardens like the Villa d'Este's makes the point that the gardens themselves are also abominations, an imposition on something already divinely ordered. Grafting falls into the same category – an unnatural use of nature.

In *Metamorphoses*, Ovid told the story of Hermaphroditus,[58] the son of Hermes and Aphrodite, drawing on the metaphor of a tree graft to present Hermaphrodite's hybridity. The story goes that Salmacis, the most beautiful of the water nymphs, was gathering lilies when she saw Hermaphroditus and had to have him. Hermaphroditus refused the nymph's advances and drove her away into the bushes. But from this undergrowth she stalked him, spying on him stripping off and paddling in the pool. She couldn't bear the sight of the naked boy, and leapt out of her hiding place, her clothes falling to the ground as she bounded towards the water and straight onto Hermaphroditus. He clung on as she twisted her body around his, literally smothering him with kisses as his head went below the water line. Gasping for air, he pleaded for his freedom, but Salmacis prayed they never be separated, and the gods heard her. The boy Hermaphroditus had always been both male and female in name – a combination of Hermes and Aphrodite – but was now a physical fusion of genders, too.

To describe this union, Ovid evoked the idea of grafting together two plants. 'As when a gardener grafts a branch on to a tree, and sees the two unite as they grow and come to maturity together,' he wrote, 'so when their limbs met in that clinging embrace the nymph and the boy were no longer two, but a single form, possessed of a dual nature, which could not be called male or female, but seemed to be at once both and neither'. Grafting in agriculture is, like the skin graft of ancient India, an extremely old procedure.

From the point of view of classical aesthetics, this dual, merged nature constituted an anomaly of nature.[59] It might even be considered abominable, monstrous. At the very least it raised questions about the nature of a grafted tree. Was it still a product of nature? In his leafy chimera, was the gardener or farmer creating something grotesque? Similar questions could be asked of the grafted bodies of Hermaphroditus and Salmacis. Were they – two bodies and two souls brought together as one – still a product of nature? Since they were no longer individuals, or even entirely male or female, did this mean they were an aberration? A transplanted tree, like a transplanted body part, is a natural form that has been tampered with and transformed into something else by human hands. What are the consequences of meddling with the natural world like this? Much like a human body, the 'disordered' wilderness was supposedly created and ordered by God and therefore not disordered at all.[60] How could any human – a gardener, in this case, but the same applies to a surgeon – dare to *improve* it? Ovid inspired gardeners for the same reason he'd eventually come to inspire those who thought about transplanting human parts, as we will soon see.

This issue of playing God was not something Tagliacozzi could ignore. He couldn't simply point out that the similarity of human skin and plant skin meant the human form could be sculpted. The human form was decidedly a product of nature – a particularly important one – and bringing a knife to it constituted an interference to that nature. His anxiety over this question was reflected in the unusual way he put together his book. If you turn past Tagliacozzi's title page, you'll find his first ten chapters have nothing to do with

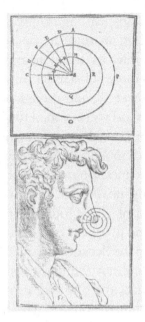

Figure 13 A Perfect Nose, images from *De Curtorum Chirurgia per Insitionem.*

grafting at all. The operation itself, in fact, accounts for a comparatively tiny proportion of the book – just the very end of it where he describes and depicts how to transplant skin. The bulk of the writing is about the dignity of the face. As if people needed convincing that losing their facial features was a horrific prospect, Tagliacozzi drew on the religious authority of the Bible and influential theologians like St Augustine and Tertullian, and appealed to the ancient authority of thinkers such as Horace, Homer and Aristotle. He sought to demonstrate the importance of the lips, ears and nose in the overall composition of the face.

By going to all this trouble, Tagliacozzi was trying to show that skin grafting was essentially a *restorative* operation. Any 'sculpting' he'd be doing had a legitimate purpose recognized in the classical and religious sources he cited. Knife-wielding tyrants and nose-dissolving diseases sliced and rotted their way through a person's face, and Tagliacozzi argued that these mutilations constituted the real damage. Grafting helped someone *reclaim* their natural proportions. He even included a handy picture to show what those proportions were, the classical idea of a perfect nose. With this evidence, Tagliacozzi was surely not inflicting further mutilation, rather conducting a salvage operation. Once a reader got as far as the operation itself, they would hopefully agree.

Although Tagliacozzi insisted that transplanting skin was nothing to fear, others would have thought that the operation did more than fiddle with the surface of the skin, and it would have pointed the way towards more substantial worries. It altered the form of a person, after all, and there *was* much to fear from tampering with God's creation. How much could a person change and still be considered a human being? At what point would they have changed so much they became an aberration, a monster? The question was one of transgressing boundaries, of smashing taxonomic categories, and of deciding what constituted playing God. These concerns, far more frightening than the prospect of a misshapen nose, would only be amplified in the decades to come. As science gave us new ways to think about the body, just around the corner in the seventeenth century would arise new, diabolical kinds of transplants: transfusions of blood would both violate our bodies and threaten to transplant more besides.

2. Blood, Animals to Animals
(1624–1665)

On 25 July 1492 Pope Innocent VIII called on his physician, Giacomo di San Genesio, and told him he was dying. Genesio saw the problem immediately: the pontiff was old. Still, the physician was convinced he could save His Holiness. He rounded up three ten-year-old Jewish boys, luring them each with a coin, then bled them dry before they could spend them. Some say the physician had Innocent drink the blood, others that the blood was transfused directly into his body. Either way, it didn't work and the pope died along with the boys.[1]

True or not, the story about Innocent VIII is the earliest reference to a (possible) blood transfusion. It demonstrates a belief in a magical link between blood and life – a bond as old as our species. Ancient Roman historian Pliny the Elder described how certain people would drink blood to make themselves younger, noting that gladiator blood was 'teeming with life' and could cure epilepsy (and that people would eat livers for the same reason). In the early twentieth century, the Scottish anthropologist J. G. Frazer also compiled in *The Golden Bough* a great many stories about blood and its universal association with life. Farmers from some cultures, he wrote, even sprinkled blood on crops so its innate life could help them grow.[2] Although blood has always been associated with life, stories about blood transfusions were rare before the seventeenth century. What few references there are tend to be sketchy on technical details, giving no real idea of how people thought blood might be taken from one body and infused into another. Under Galen's system, doctors were also more likely to relieve patients of their blood than they were to put more in, which left little medical reason to transfuse blood in the first place.

This all changed in the seventeenth century as more doctors and surgeons embraced the new trend for experimentation, valuing their own observations over the say-so of the ancients. With new ways to understand the body – ways that reflected the coming age of the machine – transfusions started to appear both possible and desirable. But with no real idea of the blood's physiological role, and since people still believed blood was infused with humours, there was no telling what effect blood transfusions might have. By the twentieth century, doctors would know much more about blood and transfusion would have an essential role in modern transplant surgery. But in the seventeenth century, budding transfusionists thought such transferral might be useful in other ways and competition broke out between France and England, as religious tensions and outrage erupted amongst those who saw transfusion as beneficial and those who saw it as unnatural, unnecessary and dangerous. By today's standards, no seventeenth-century transfusion was successful. But some of the most highly regarded doctors and surgeons at the time were convinced that, by breaching the previously unbroken barrier between two bodies, transfusing blood might, as the legends say, be the key to a long life and everlasting youth.

The Origins of Spare-Part Surgery

When William Harvey walked through the Gate of Honour at Caius College with a BA in medicine at the very end of the sixteenth century, the medical system was still dominated by Galen.[3] But Harvey was a physician with a double life. By day, he was a good, Galenic teacher. He followed in the footsteps of John Caius, graduating from the University of Padua in 1602, then immediately starting work at St Bartholomew's Hospital, where Caius had died nearly thirty years earlier. By night, however, he took his lead from Caius's opponent, Vesalius, on a quest to discover all he could about the heart. And he spent much of the late 1610s and early 1620s slicing them up.

One evening at his dissection table, he cut open the body of a hanged man acquired from another of Caius's old haunts, the College of Physicians. He cracked open the thorax, exposed the heart, then tied shut the pulmonary artery and injected water into the right ventricle. Any of his students would have been able to parrot what he taught them – that the blood would pass through pores in the septum to allow blood to mingle with air. They would have expected the water to seep from one ventricle to the other, but as Harvey's hand worked a syringe stuck into the right ventricle, it got larger and larger, inflating like a balloon until it threatened to burst. Not a drop passed over to the left ventricle, which remained inert, as if emphasizing its swollen counterpart. Here was proof there were no pores in the septum. As the right ventricle collapsed back into itself and Harvey turned away from the carcass, he knew the necessary next stage of his research would be to observe the motion of a heart in vivo.

Experimenting on living humans was out of the question, so Harvey went after London's aquatic life and netted a shrimp from the Thames. Holding a magnifying glass up to its belly, he could see right through its transparent shell to its heart. He saw it expanding and contracting, convinced he could see the blood leaving the heart when it contracted. But a shrimp is tiny, its heartbeat fast, so he couldn't be sure. Wading around in the Thames some more, he got hold of a large fish, took it home and slapped it down on his table. While it was still wriggling, he sliced into its body and hovered a finger over its still-beating heart. In the short time before it died, he felt the heart alternating from soft to hard, repeatedly, soft to hard. It behaved, he saw, like a muscle. To confirm his point, he also sliced a live eel in two, scooped out and scrutinized its heart, which in his hands became a disembodied mass of muscular contractions.

The next animal Harvey tied, face-up, to his sacrificial table was a whimpering dog. He drove his knife into its chest. Stretching open the skin flaps, he found what he was looking for – blood entering the heart on the right side via the vena cava and exiting again through the pulmonary artery. Peering into the still-alive, agonized animal, he carefully noted how its blood flowed up to the lungs and back into the heart, but this time in the left ventricle via the pulmonary vein. From there, the blood circulated the entire system of the animal, which, by the time Harvey was making these observations, was writhing in sync with its faltering heart. These grizzly evenings with scalpel in hand paid off, including the times when he took his knife to his own dead father and sister. Not only was Galen's anatomy wrong – something Vesalius had already started to show – but he also had the wrong idea about how the blood and heart worked.

In Galen's traditional account, the body produced blood to order. Each body part behaved as if it had a mind of its own, starting with the stomach-hand reaching up the gullet to grab the food. The liver would then transform this food – 'concoct' it – into blood. The rest of the body would attract this blood when it was needed, to heal or to grow. The lungs and brain would also draw some of it to themselves and infuse it with their respective 'vital' and 'psychic' spirits. But this, Harvey found, must all be wrong. The anatomist's observations showed that the heart *pumped* blood from part to part, so it continually circulated. The heart, he calculated, beat about 2,000 times in an hour, so roughly 2,000 drachms (about 7.1 litres) would have to pass through it during this time. If blood was produced and consumed directly, as in Galen's elaborate account, the liver would have to manufacture around 50,000 drachms, or nearly 180 litres, in a day, which would surely be impossible. Even if Harvey's guesstimates were a little inaccurate, the intellectual argument still stood: livers clearly couldn't produce anywhere near so much blood.

You can try one of Harvey's less lethal experiments on yourself. First, tie a ligature around your arm. It will obstruct your blood flow, and you'll notice a 'tidal swell', to use Harvey's description, as if your blood is trying to burst through the blockage. After a while, your hand will start to cool and get paler. Once you loosen the ligature, your hand will flush red with a large amount of blood as if a dam had burst. Your arm will feel warm and pulsate with each beat of your heart. It's an uncomfortable but effective way of taking the idea of circulation beyond a disembodied theory, to feel the throbbing of your blood as your heart propels it around your body.

The heart as a pump is now a go-to and even clichéd metaphor, but for Harvey it was a revelation. It meant he could appreciate the body – at least this part – as if it was a mechanism. He lectured about, and demonstrated, the circulation of the blood from about 1615, and in 1624 published his discovery in Latin. Then in 1628 it came out in English. When Harvey likened the heart and circulatory system to a pump and the vena cava to 'the cellar and cistern of the blood', he dragged the body out of an agricultural frame and into a mechanical

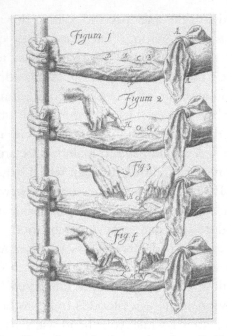

Figure 14 William Harvey's experiments on the valves, *De Motu Cordis*, 1628.

one. Microscopes, telescopes and pendulum clocks started to spring up about this time, too, captivating us and inviting us to relate to the world in novel ways. Reflecting a new fashion for and fascination with gadgets like these, people started to look at their bodies anew.

The revolutionary idea – that body parts were like mechanical components – quickly gained traction through the seventeenth century, even during Harvey's own lifetime. The poet John Donne – the man who wrote that 'no man is an island' – was an early adopter. In 1621 he wrote a sermon referring to the 'conduits and cisterns of the body', an image some historians think may have come from Harvey's lectures.[4] By 1637, René Descartes was likening the 'nature of the bloud' with 'the motions of a clock' and its 'weight and wheels'.[5] Twenty-four years later, the Italian biologist Marcello Malpighi turned the relatively new technology of the microscope onto the body to observe blood flowing 'in a tortuous path and in different directions' through tiny networks of vessels.[6] These capillaries joined the venous and arterial systems – a mechanism Harvey had deduced but had never seen for himself. Malpighi extended Harvey's machine metaphor even further: from his *Anatome Plantarum* we learned that the body is a loom, weaving together not only vegetable matter but also bones and teeth.[7] And Charles Le Brun, in 1668, in his *Conférence sur l'Expression* – a book about the science of passions and emotional expressions – called the eyebrows the 'motor of the face', expressing how even emotions were, when it came down to it, mechanical.[8]

Seventeenth-century doctors, surgeons and philosophers could interpret their bodies in the mechanical language of their age. They saw pumps, looms, clocks, cisterns, pulleys and even rudimentary cameras where they once saw apple and pear trees. The body was on the way to being a machine in every regard. It behaved, like any other kind of engine, according to reason. Mechanists proudly held up their hearts, engines of their bodies, circulators of their blood. It would take a few decades before anyone dared openly dispense with God as a prime mover, but during these few years at the start of the seventeenth century, it became conceivable that a skilled medical practitioner could take a broken body part and either fix it or replace it entirely. These were, in other words, the origins of spare-part surgery.

But there was another side to the discipline. For the majority of early mechanists, a body of spare parts was still animated by a divine soul or spirit. This was true even for

Harvey himself. He may have been one of the architects of modern medicine, clarifying the heart's function as a mere pump, but he still referred to that pump as 'the seat and organ of all passions'.[9] In his dedication in *De Motu Cordis*, too, he embraced old-fashioned microcosm–macrocosm relationships, associating the body with other structures (the state, for example, and even the heavens and the seasons). 'Most illustrious King!' he wrote in his dedication to the monarch, 'the animal's heart is the basis of its life, its chief member, the sun of its microcosm; on the heart all its activity depends, from the heart all its liveliness and strength arise'. He goes on to explain how the king fulfils the same role in the body of the state. Here Harvey compared the heart to the monarch. Flattery it may have been, but it's also an intellectual move familiar to classically trained physicians. Galen was another physician who saw the world in a grain of sand and heaven in a flower when he lined up the human body with the four humours, temperaments and seasons, and saw it all in relation to the stars.

For a supposedly modern man, Harvey's ideas are laced with mystery, magical beliefs and ancient classical ideas. But that's because he wasn't a modern man. He certainly wouldn't have described himself in this way. He in fact had a special name for doctors he considered to be modern: 'shitt-breeches'.[10] He preferred to recommend his colleagues go straight to 'the fountainhead' of the ancients – Aristotle, Cicero, Avicenna. Even when he devised some of his thought experiments, like measuring the amount of blood passing through the heart, Harvey was directly inspired by Aristotle, who'd used a similar formula to explain the water cycle in nature: the world didn't contain enough water for it to flow from the top of the mountain and into the sea without there being some way to get it back up to the top again. It was a set of classical philosophers and physicians that helped Harvey explain the importance of blood, and how our bodies are 'nourished, warmed, and activated' by it.

So, yes, blood was pumped around the body. Yes, it behaved according to reason. But, for Harvey, it was also magical; nothing less than a vehicle of 'natural, powerful, fiery heat'. It was 'a sort of store of life', he wrote, 'impregnated with spirits'.[11] We think of Descartes – the philosopher who wrote 'I think therefore I am' – as similarly modern because he, too, embraced mechanisms and was directly inspired by Harvey. But he also thought 'the weights and wheels' of the body were moved by 'animall spirits', which were 'a most subtil wind . . . a most pure and lively flame'.[12] Sometimes it's hard to distinguish between the ancient and the modern.

Even now, when the physiological role of the blood is no longer such a secret, we still convince ourselves about the truth and significance of long-discredited ideas. We have family blood, national blood, and embrace this kind of talk as we construct ideas about ourselves and identify with our tribes. Thinking about blood in this way began as an attempt at explaining how the world really works and has since been reduced – or elevated – to poetry. Elevated because traditions still have meaning and they influence the way we think about ourselves and our relationships with one another. Times have changed, but we've brought the cultural weight of the blood with us.

The same is true of our family names. Most cultures take their fathers' last names. They do this out of tradition and because for millennia they've been taught about the innate superiority of men over women. For the likes of Aristotle and Galen, as we have seen, this was a biological fact, since they thought sperm formed the hard, permanent bits of the body – the organs and bones – which gave form to the other squishy bits, created directly from the instruction-taking menstrual blood.[13] We now accept men aren't inherently biologically 'superior', but it's still conventional for wives to take their husband's name, and even children of unmarried parents are frequently given their fathers' surnames, as if it's the male 'blood line' that gives literal shape to the family.

Similarly, people from many cultures wear wedding rings on the finger next to the little finger, most often on the left hand. We do this because under the Galenic, humoral system of medicine the blood vessels in that finger led straight to the heart. This is true, but we now know that *every* blood vessel leads to the heart. There's no reason to single out the ring finger any more, no reason to push a ring onto it. But we do it anyway.

This human reticence to change is perhaps also why, when Harvey discovered the circulation of the blood, he found his experiments were bad for business. Even though he was a superb anatomist, the biographer John Aubrey wrote, no one would give three shillings for one of his prescriptions (and even if they did, he bitched, they wouldn't have been able to read his scrawl[14]). Harvey held the prestigious Lumleian lectureship at the College of Physicians, and was even Physician Extraordinary to James I, but his new-fangled ways frightened off patients, who sought comfort in the old ways of traditional doctors. The anatomist nevertheless won his fair share of admirers and by 1632 became Physician in Ordinary to Charles I. So at least in royalist circles his reputation was secured.

With this human tendency to cling to old ways in mind, it's perhaps easier to understand how even some of the most enlightened doctors of the seventeenth century would have planted only one foot in the modern world, leaving the other with the ancients. When Harvey had just discovered circulation, rather than rip up their books, some physicians made links to their traditional systems. You'd think phlebotomy, for example, would have gone out of the window along with Galen, but physicians simply crammed Harvey's theory into existing models.[15] They convinced themselves that because blood constantly circulates, it was of even greater importance than they first thought. So, they assigned to it many of the properties they'd previously ascribed to other humours and bled their patients still more.

Thus, although we might think about modern ideas like circulation as killing off the ancient ones like vitalism and humoralism, this wasn't the case. To make sense of the mystery of the blood, people combined what they knew of the body's mechanism with the old Galenic system and any other beliefs they happened to hold. For a few brief years to come, and for a few eccentric visionaries, Galen and the new mechanist philosophy, represented in medicine by Harvey, even made sense together. Old and new mingled. It was from a combination of those medical systems – along with a dollop of religion and superstition – that blood transfusion first emerged, promising the world and threatening a chaos rivalling anything Ovid ever conjured.

The First Blood Transfusion

While Harvey was busying himself with his corpses in the 1620s, King Charles I had dissolved three Parliaments. And he ruled without Parliament at all in the so-called Eleven Years' Tyranny blotting the 1630s. In a final series of crises, Parliament was recalled to raise money for a war with Scotland, the

Irish rose against English rule and Charles attempted to arrest his political opponents. After nearly two decades of upheaval, Harvey's patron raised his royal standard in Nottingham in 1642, and both sovereign and Parliament rallied their respective royalist and parliamentarian supporters for war. By the end of October – just two months later – William Harvey was at the battle of Edgehill, discharging his duty protecting Charles I's children: Prince James and the future Charles II.[16]

Throughout the turbulent 1640s, Harvey's commitment to science never wavered. He continued to influence the story of mechanical medicine, and two strains of research in particular that brought about the first blood transfusions. One individual, Francis Potter, was responsible for the first.[17] Potter was a clergyman, best known now for his book *Interpretation of the Number 666*, written in 1642,[18] and for claiming the Pope was the Antichrist. Harvey had business at Trinity College, Oxford studying the embryological development of hens' eggs with his friend Ralph Bathurst and would stop by to see Potter whenever he was around.[19] As well as being a clergyman, Potter was also an inventor and enjoyed building machines. One of these – a pulley system designed to heave an unusually heavy bucket from a deep well – attracted the praise of the biographer John Aubrey, who also became one of Potter's closest friends. Given Harvey's history cutting open human machinery, the circulatory system was doubtless amongst the mechanical topics the two men discussed.

It was around the same time that Potter started to ponder the tale of Jason and the Argonauts from Ovid's *Metamorphoses*. In this story Jason, leader of the Minyans, set sail up the River Phasis in search of the golden fleece, which the king agreed Jason could have, but only if he performed some daring tasks. First, he had to yoke and plough a field with fire-breathing bulls, then into that field plant dragon's teeth and defeat the legion of fully armed men that grew from them. Once he'd done that, he finally had to steal the fleece itself from under the nose of a sleepless, fork-tongued dragon. As the king posed his challenges, his daughter, Medea, swiftly fell in love with the hero and deployed her magic so that when Jason confronted the bulls he couldn't feel the flames licking at him, and when the army spawned from the ground, her magic helped him confuse and defeat them. And as Jason squared up to the sleepless dragon, her magical drugs sent it into the first slumber it had ever known. It was Medea's magic, and what happened next, that occupied Potter's thoughts for many years.

Jason claimed both the fleece and Medea herself, and with the rest of his company they sailed back to Thessaly to be greeted by the liberal burning of incense, an animal sacrifice and jubilant fathers celebrating the return of their sons. Only Jason's father, it seemed, was not present. He was too aged and feeble to come out of his house. Recalling how his new wife had helped him with his own impossible tasks, Jason pleaded with tears in his eyes that she call on her god-given magic to take some years from his own lifespan and give them to his father.

Jason's plea moved Medea, but she wouldn't countenance shortening her husband's life. She agreed to extend his father's life in another way, 'with the help not of your years', she said, 'but of my skill'. So, she hopped onto a chariot pulled by flying dragons, and for nine days and nine nights soared around the known world collecting rare and precious ingredients including moonlight, frost, pieces of owl, tortoises, wolves, stags, and the face and beak of an elderly crow. Winging her way back to Thessaly, she concocted her potion and performed a dark ritual involving the blood of a ram and fire.

She had the frail frame of Jason's father brought out and laid upon a carpet of herbs. At the opportune moment, she slit his throat. As the aged blood streamed out of the wound and down his neck, she replaced it with her youth-giving potion, making him drink some of it and putting the rest directly into his body through the wound (in some versions of Medea's story, her potion is first mixed with the spilled blood, which is then sent back into the old man's body). With the vitalizing blood now rejuvenating his body, Jason's father started to transform. His white hair darkened, his papery skin plumped out, pinking up as time was reversed and he became once more a young man.[20]

Jason and the Argonauts featured no surgery as such. It did, however, like many of Ovid's stories, describe a chaotic world where flesh is not the boundary we believe it to be. On an intuitive level, the idea that you could create unnatural connections between two bodies invests the concepts of transplantation and transfusion with all kinds of possibilities. Given the dominance of the Galenic system of medicine, it wasn't so far-fetched to think that a blood transfusion might make a recipient younger, or prompt some other seemingly outlandish transformation. Classical medicine showed just how everyday, benign and gradual metamorphosis could be. Considering how digestion was seen as a transformation of plant into person, a metamorphosis could be as unthreatening as eating a lettuce. And if you believed that metamorphosis is the natural way of things, it would be far easier to accept the possibility of other transformations. Potter wondered if transfusion would be feasible in the real world.

As it happens, earlier in the century, in 1615, the German

physician Andreas Libavius had already contemplated transfusing blood. He imagined it would be a case of moving life
from a young, 'robust' man to an old, emaciated one, pictur-
ing a man so old he could hardly keep his soul in his body.
There's no evidence he actually tried it, but if only you could
move the younger person's blood into the older one's body,
he thought, the old man would start to recuperate the strength
of his earlier years, just like Jason's father had. Libavius
thought blood was filled with spirit, with life itself, and he
wrote about transfusion as if a young human body could
become a fountain of life, its vitalizing fluids distributed into
an older soul. He closed his book, however, with a statement
about how foolish it would be to try this in real life.

Potter was not a great reader, so – according to Aubrey, who
name-checks Libavius – he probably hadn't heard about the
German's musings on transfusion. He had, though, been having weekly chats with William Harvey, and knew about the
circulation of the blood – an advantage not shared by Libavius,
who was writing even before this discovery. If there was such a
thing as a circulatory system, Potter mused, it should be possible to interrupt that system and insert some fluid into it.
Getting blood from one body to another would just be a matter
of ingenuity, the application of a practical mind, a mechanistic
mind such as his own. Then, in an example of the new world
of machines meeting the old world, Potter thought it might be
possible to magically cure all sorts of diseases and conditions if
he could overcome the mechanical challenge.

By the time he finally decided to try out his idea, the Civil
War had disturbed Potter's well-ordered world in Oxford. The
mid-1640s were particularly rough for royalists. Between 1646
and 1647 Charles I had surrendered to the Scottish, and Cromwell's New Model Army laid siege to – then marched into and

took – Oxford. After the siege, Potter withdrew to settle in the rectory at Kilmington, then in Somerset, about halfway between Bristol and Bournemouth. He reputedly lived a mostly solitary life, snipping away at the hedges in his garden and dedicating time to building mechanical devices in his private laboratory. Aubrey visited him, and in his *Brief Lives* described him as the man 'most like a monk' he'd ever seen, even living in a house so sparsely decorated that it resembled a monastic cell, though peppered with his 'many ingenious inventions'.

Aubrey also joined Potter for what might have been his first transfusion experiment, recalling how in 1650 they tried to collect blood from one hen to inject into another. But they hit two problems. First, they had difficulty drawing the blood in the first place, and second, it tended to clot while they were fiddling about with tiny ivory pipes and tubes to prepare the recipient animal. 'The creature [was] too little', reflected Aubrey, 'and our tooles not good.'[21] The biographer seems to have left Potter to it, sending him a surgeon's lancet in the post and a note encouraging him to carry on trying.

A couple of years later, Aubrey got another letter from Potter, who was keen to tell him how he'd progressed. To more effectively collect the blood, he was now using a pair of miniature bellows. And he'd replaced the ivory pipe with the windpipe of a 'small animal'. But he could never quite get it to work and his experiment sank into obscurity. It was not the last time a mechanically minded man would attempt to harness the mysterious power within the blood, though. The second strain of research Harvey's work had set in motion had greater longevity. It involved a more organized group of scientists and doctors who would eventually become part of the Royal Society, still in existence today.

While in Oxford, Harvey got to know a royalist soldier

called Charles Scarburgh,[22] who would later become a doctor with such singular skill the poet Abraham Cowley honoured him in an ode: 'Scarce could the Sword dispatch more to the Grave', Cowley enthused, 'Than Thou didst save.' By the time he was sixty-nine, Scarburgh was considered so reliable as a doctor that he attended – and took overall responsibility for the treatment of – Charles II in his final, fatal illness. Before the war he'd been studying, like many of his predecessors, at Caius College in Cambridge. But Cambridge was one of the first cities to fall to parliamentary forces, and the royalist Scarburgh fled to join the king's army in Oxford, where he met and befriended Harvey. Harvey was so impressed with his young acquaintance that later, from London, he wrote hoping to convince Scarburgh to 'leave off gunning' and join him in the medical profession. When Oxford came under siege, Scarburgh slipped out of that city as he had Cambridge, probably paying a fine, or 'compound', to the occupying forces to guarantee his freedom. He took Harvey's advice, and with MD in hand, settled in London as a physician.

In the meantime, the Scottish sold the king back to his parliamentarian enemies. As their world collapsed around them, it was around Scarburgh's dinner table that top royalist intellectuals gathered. Many had directly served the king as physicians and, like Scarburgh himself, this select group were well versed in William Harvey's circulation ideas. One of the group's core members, George Ent, had written a whole book – *Apologia Pro Circulatione Sanguinis* – in defence of Harvey. Another, Nathaniel Highmore, was soon (in 1651) to publish an entire anatomical textbook incorporating his theory. It's thanks to this war – and Scarburgh's dinner parties – that the Royal Society eventually formed, and early scientists stared to get to grips with the circulatory system as a mechanism they might be able to use for medical purposes. It was here that the seeds of the first sustained research programme into blood transfusion were sown.

One day Scarburgh welcomed to his table a young man from a well-known royalist family who would become instrumental in early blood transfusion: Christopher Wren. The Great Fire of London and the architectural commission that would make his name – the redesign of St Paul's Cathedral – were a few years away yet. At just fifteen, Wren, a sickly child, came to Scarburgh as a patient. The two got along, and Wren became first his pupil and then his assistant. Over the next couple of years, he also found a friend in Scarburgh, as well as a master teacher of mathematics and medicine, and someone to introduce him to a group of other philosophers, doctors and mathematicians. These would be important contacts now that Charles I had been executed, and the country newly reconstituted a republic in January 1649. One of Wren's early opportunities through Scarburgh and his many contacts was to translate into Latin a slim tract on sundials for mathematician William Oughtred, published in 1652. His work was so well received he was appointed to a fellowship at All Soul's College in Oxford – a nomination all the more exceptional in parliamentarian Oxford since Wren's father had been chaplain to the king and had even refused to give up the keys of the chapel when the parliamentarians invaded Windsor Castle.

When some members of Scarburgh's circle started to gather in Oxford in the 1650s, they instituted a more formal structure to their meetings, along with a deliberate research programme. Since science and the pursuit of knowledge must, as a matter of principle, be impartial, Scarburgh's royalist group clubbed together with parliamentarian scientists.

'The Ruines of a Civil War thou dost alone repair', wrote Abraham Cowley in his ode to Scarburgh, probably referring to the social 'wounds' healed at his dinner table. The new group professed neutrality, rallying not around religion or political loyalty, but rather the spirit exemplified by Harvey and his ideas, which had by now not only been generally accepted but were also being taught in medical schools all over Europe. Though he seems to have played no direct part in transfusing blood, Scarburgh fulfilled an important role in putting Wren in touch with this new social circle, and with two men in particular.

John Wilkins, the warden of Wadham College, Oxford, became something of a nucleus for the group and joined Wren in some early investigations. Wilkins's parliamentarian credentials were so strong he even married Oliver Cromwell's youngest sister. But in the non-partisan, nurturing bosom of those who now called themselves the 'Invisible College', Wilkins became another mentor to the royalist Wren. He was also probably the man who arranged his professorship in astronomy at Gresham College in London in August 1657. (Wren was actually supposed to take a chair in geology, but Laurence Rooke, the sitting professor of astronomy, wanted the bigger apartment and balcony that came with the geology professorship, so he arranged to move sideways, despite not being a geologist, and Wren made do with Rooke's old digs on Broad Street.) Joining Wren and Wilkins was Robert Boyle. Boyle is today lauded as the first modern chemist, famous for suffocating birds in his air pump to study respiration, amongst many other experiments. Since his loyalty was divided – his father being royalist and his sister parliamentarian – he fitted in well with the Invisible College.

It was Boyle's curiosity that led the others along the path

towards transfusion. He wanted to puzzle out how a person could be incapacitated by an abscess that only appeared in their hand or leg. How could a local wound impact an entire body? He first conducted some experiments alone, feeding the head, tail and gall of a viper to a dog – the parts of a snake that people thought contained the venom. In *De Motu Cordis*, Harvey had remarked, as one of his proofs of circulation constantly taking place in the body, that poisons and medicines must circulate with the blood. And the body was supposed to convert food straight into blood, so it made sense the toxins would get into the bloodstream this way. The dog gobbled up the snake parts, and Boyle watched, expecting the poison to make its way to the bloodstream. But nothing out of the ordinary happened. The dog continued to wag its tail and Boyle continued to scratch his head.[23]

His next thought was that a snake bite might be deadly because there was something in its anger. Since no one yet understood rabies, this made sense, too, because when a mad dog goes into a rage, its bite causes 'a nasty illness'. Dogs aren't venomous, so it made sense that the toxins might have come about through the rage itself. And he speculated that he might cover a needle in venom and insert it into a dog, to see whether it was the venom or the anger.[24] In Boyle's mind here was a basic kind of infusion, but he never got around to trying it, until he met Christopher Wren.

It was 1656. Boyle had only just moved to Oxford that year, and he was squirrelled away in his lodgings with Wilkins and Wren. He summoned a 'large dog' from somewhere and sent for Thomas Willis (a pioneer of brain research) and John Bathurst (Oliver Cromwell's physician). He later recalled tying the 'tortured animal' to the table, binding each leg to a corner and preparing a syringe with some opium dissolved in sack (fortified wine). Hypodermic needles such as the ones we're familiar with today did not exist until the mid-nineteenth century, so using a syringe required the scientists to uncover and make an incision directly into a large vessel. With the opium administered, the men could barely untie all four of the dog's limbs before the solution took effect.

Immediately, the dog nodded his head and reeled around, high as a kite. It was an uncertain few minutes as Boyle whipped it up and down his garden to keep it awake. The rest of the group placed bets on whether it would ultimately survive being shot up with opium. It did survive. Boyle took it in, nursed it back to health over the coming days and made it a canine celebrity. But the now-famous creature was soon dognapped. Boyle, Wilkins and Wren had, however, become the first to observe what happened when substances rode the bloodstream directly to the brain. They repeated the experiment again and again, hoping to find out more about this quicker, more direct way to get substances into the body than swallowing and digesting them. When they injected dogs with opiates, they got high quicker; when they administered emetics, they vomited sooner; and when they gave them alcohol, they got drunk earlier but 'soon after pisseth it out'. And they didn't need as much of the substance in question for it to be effective.[25]

Eventually they refined their equipment and replaced the syringe with a bladder attached to a hollowed-out goose or porcupine quill. By filling this bladder with the drugs or alcohol, they could squeeze the substances through the quill, directly into the bloodstream. William Harvey was still alive, though approaching the end of his seventies, when Wren, Boyle and Wilkins performed these experiments. What started life as Harvey's mental fidget, likening the circulatory system to a machine, this curious set of scientists took seriously. For the history of transplantation, they were a significant step because the quill acted as the world's first effective mechanical substitute for a body part – in this case, a blood vessel. Other transfusion researchers would use different materials. The French transfusionist Jean-Baptiste Denis used silver pipes. Robert Hooke – an early adopter of microscopy, Boyle's assistant and Wren's best friend – suggested brass pipes.[26] Italian transfusionists would later, in the 1660s, even experiment with glass tubes. When researchers saw these makeshift mechanical blood vessels working, they not only took them as evidence that living things are machines, but also as proof that bits of one creature could be replaced by bits of another.

On 26 June 1657, just a few months later, William Harvey's body set out on a fifty-mile-long funeral procession from London to Hempstead in Essex. The grand old doctor had died of a cerebral haemorrhage twenty-three days earlier at the age of seventy-nine. His corpse was encased in lead – a practice John Aubrey described as peculiar to the Harvey family – as friends and enrobed members of the College of Physicians conveyed him to St Andrew's Church. Many of those accompanying Harvey's leaden sarcophagus had been remembered by the grand physician, either materially or with career-making favour. Scarburgh was beneficiary of both. He inherited Harvey's velvet gown and 'little silver instruments of surgerie', landed a job at St Bartholomew's Hospital on Harvey's recommendation, and succeeded him as Lumleian lecturer. Harvey's final journey would have taken a few days, but the more important mourners would have peeled off at some point the first morning – Oliver Cromwell was being inaugurated for the second time, back in London.[27]

With Harvey's body at rest in Hempstead, Wren moved to

London and got in touch with an old friend, Timothy Clarke, another doctor he'd met in Oxford. Together, they started to run yet more injection experiments until August 1657, when they decided it was time to move on from animals and inject a human. Boyle wrote about the episode a few years later.[28] The French ambassador to the Commonwealth had an 'inferior' domestic servant, he wrote, who 'deserv'd to have been hang'd'. He didn't write why he deserved to have been hanged, but this became their man, the first human being to be injected intravenously and given an armful of an emetic called *crocus metallorum*. At least, that was the plan. Wren and Clarke restrained him, like one of the dogs in their earlier experiments, and the man broke, either fainting or pretending to faint. They called off the whole experiment.

Members of both Oxford and London circles continued experimenting with injection over the coming years, and into the Restoration that came in 1660. What started as Charles Scarburgh's learned dinner parties was finally established as a formal society in 1660.[29] They held their first official meeting after one of Wren's Gresham College lectures at the end of November that year. The boy that William Harvey had watched over at the Battle of Edgehill was now King Charles II, and the monarch confirmed the 'Royal' bit of the Royal Society in 1662. Boyle, Wilkins and Wren were amongst the first fellows, as was the Ovid-inspired Francis Potter, who was admitted in November 1663. The Royal Society's motto, *Nullius in verba*, means 'take nobody's word for it'. It reflected an approach to knowledge that characterized the new science and medicine, and its commitment to establishing fact through experimentation and empiricism. As Fioravanti, Vesalius and Harvey all did in their own ways, the fellows trusted only what they could see with their own eyes and sense with their own senses.

The newly incorporated Royal Society was getting closer to performing the first blood transfusion. Boyle had been receiving letters from an outsider, a physician called Richard Lower who had been a student at Oxford with Wren. In one of his letters, Lower told Boyle about a fancy he had to see 'how long a dog may live without meat, by syringing into a vein a due quantity of good broth'. He proposed injecting food directly into the bloodstream, and promised he'd get a two-inch tin pipe made, 'about the usual bigness of a jugular vein', and try it. A year later he injected two quarts of spa water from Tunbridge Wells into a dog. He hoped he'd notice its reputed healing properties on another one of seventeenth-century England's long-suffering dog population, but the only effect seems to have been that the dog, as he put it, 'discharged itself'. He later wrote another letter wondering if it would be possible to fix a pipe permanently into a dog so he could now and then shovel food into it. There is no evidence he ever did this. If he had, he would have created a rudimentary intravenous drip. A couple of years later, however, in 1664, he had another go at feeding a dog directly through its bloodstream. He prepared his syringe with milk this time, and injected two pints of it. The dog died within the hour. When Lower dragged his scalpel through the vessels, he found them clogged up with a curd of blood and milk.[30] It must have been a painful death for the poor dog, but it turned out to be an important moment because it highlighted how complicated blood was, and how tricky it was to work with. If he wanted to feed an animal intravenously, he'd need to have another think about compatibility – how to stop the blood from clotting and curdling.

His next move made him the first transfusionist (unless you include Francis Potter's unsuccessful dabblings). If the dog digested the milk in the normal way – that was, after drinking it – he reasoned, it would have ended up in the blood-stream, so he could try taking the blood from one dog and giving it to another. To test whether this had a chance of working, he sloshed the bloods of different animals together in another experiment and noticed they 'mingled freely'. There didn't seem to be any bad reactions. But he did notice that blood tended to coagulate outside the body, which meant he couldn't put it in a syringe. Thinking like a good mechanist, he wrote that getting blood from one body into another would be a 'simple' matter of extending 'the first animal's circulation'.

So, he tried this, laying dogs side by side, making the necessary incisions, variously connecting veins to veins and arteries to arteries, using hollow reeds and tin pipes in place of Wren's porcupine quills and Potter's windpipe. For a year his experiments always ended with a thin dribble of blood that caked up before it got out of the donor's body – a problem Potter and Aubrey had come up against earlier in the century. He got no further until he worked out that he needed to connect arteries to veins to make use of the pumping action of the heart. So, he laid two creatures side by side again, pulled out their vessels – one artery and one vein – lined them up, and put a tube between them. Using this method, the blood flowed more freely, the arterial flow actively propelling the liquid through the connecting mechanism. For a short time, the two dogs had a single circulatory system, blood travelling from one body to the other. In a sense, they became, albeit temporarily, one animal. Here, for the first time in the history of transplantation, we have something like a donor–recipient relationship: two creatures involved in the same transaction of body parts. But it would be anachronistic to use the terms 'donor' and 'recipient' as we understand them today. His dog certainly wasn't 'donating', and the 'recipient' had no reason to be thankful.

Lower himself described one as 'emitting', the other 'receiving'[31] – cold terms that betray a mechanist's attitude towards animals and to blood. Cutting up animals and experimenting on their internal organs while they were still alive was not new in the seventeenth century – Aristotle, Galen and many others had conducted their own experiments over the preceding centuries. But to speak of living beings as if they were machine parts was new. Descartes, who, after hearing about circulation, was quick to compare animals to clocks and pulley systems, thought animals couldn't feel pain. The philosopher separated the mind from the body, and animals had no mind. As mere machines, they were simply incapable of any kind of emotional response. Thinking and feeling, in fact, were reserved exclusively for human beings. Anything you might take as an expression of pain from an animal, he thought, was really just a consequence of matter acting upon matter. Although Lower would almost certainly have known Descartes's position, there is no record that he ever mentioned the French philosopher in relation to his animal subjects – none of the early English transfusionists seem to have.[32]

In fact, it was apparently very rare for *anyone* to bring up his 'beast-machine' justification directly. Despite being a modern scientist, Robert Boyle – who was one of the most prodigious experimenters on live animals – adopted an ancient philosophical justification: humankind has dominion over other living things. It was even Christian, he suggested, to conduct what would now be called vivisections. God gave humans 'that noble faculty called reason', he wrote, and it was their responsibility to dissect God's creation, understand it and figure out how best to use it. Motivated by this excuse, he suffocated sparrows, larks, mice, ducks and cats in his vacuum pump. During experiments on the respiratory system, he once tried to drown a duck before the Society, lifting it out of the water every now and then to check if it was dead. The diarist and gardener John Evelyn sat in on one of Boyle's dissections, and admitted it was too cruel for his taste. And Boyle's own assistant, Robert Hooke, confided that when he experimented on animals, he felt sorry for them, and wondered whether it would be possible to 'stupefy' them before their dissections (but there was no opiate strong enough to ease the animal's pain). Boyle had at least one soft spot: he only ever suffocated one kitten. He brought a second to the edge of death in one experiment and was planning to make it repeat its ordeal, but something tugged at his heartstrings and he admitted that would be 'too severe'.[33]

Whether or not he engaged with Descartes's theory, Lower certainly treated animal bodies as mere machines. Not only did this mean he would pull the poor creatures apart without taking any notice of their anguished howls, it also guided the direction of his experiments, working out how to move fluids

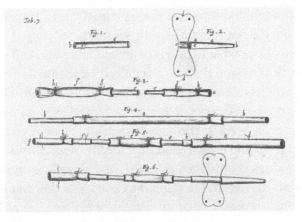

Figure 15 Richard Lower's transfusion equipment, 1666.

from one receptacle to another. Transfusion was, for him, a matter of emptying and filling animal bodies. He even spent days thinking about filling up different sizes of dogs, using lots of smaller dogs to fill up a big dog, and one giant dog to supply an entire pack of puppies. At this stage in its history, blood transfusion was a mechanical problem, nothing more.

At a meeting of the Royal Society in February 1665,[34] the pioneering Lower finally performed his transfusion experiment for an audience. As he uncoupled the two creatures, he explained that one animal could live with the blood of another. He even went so far as to say that sheep blood might agree with humans and so could be a remedy for patients who'd suffered severe blood loss. In the spirit promoted by the Royal Society – *Nullius in verba* – Lower also explained how he'd tried exchanging the blood of 'old and young, sick and healthy, hot and cold, fierce and fearful, tame and wild animals'. But, in contrast to the magical cure of diseases that Potter had hoped to find years earlier, he found that an animal's 'nature or disposition' made no difference to the outcome of the experiment.

After this momentous demonstration, Robert Boyle wondered where blood transfusion might go next. In January 1666 he read out a list of sixteen investigations in a meeting. Amongst questions about what happens to an animal's pulse and urine, it seemed Boyle wanted more structured experiments on nutrition. If you feed one dog then transfuse its blood into a hungry dog, would the recipient no longer be hungry? Could you keep a dog alive by feeding through transfusion? Could you cure a sick dog by giving it the blood of a healthy dog? He also asked how the dogs themselves changed, and what was transfused along with the blood. He wanted to know whether transfusion altered the 'disposition' of an animal, 'whether a *fierce* Dog by being often new stocked with the blood of a *cowardly* Dog, may not be more tame'. Would a dog know its master and remember any tricks it had been taught? Would a small dog stocked with the blood of a big dog grow in size? An old dog get younger? Would the 'hair or feathers' of a recipient animal change colour to that of the emittant? And what effect will transfusion have on the offspring of pregnant recipients?[35]

Over the next couple of years, other members of the Royal Society would repeat Lower's experiments for an audience. In one performed by Edmund King and Thomas Coxe and attended by the diarist Samuel Pepys, a mastiff 'emitted' the blood, a spaniel 'received' it. The two scientists arranged the experiment this way because a dog with a slower heart rate made its blood flow easier to manage. In his diary, Pepys wrote it up as a 'pretty experiment'. But when all the spectators had gone home, the scientists noted over the next few days that, although the mastiff had died, the spaniel seemed to put on a lot of weight, getting bigger and fatter. It was almost as if the heft of the mastiff had somehow transferred itself into the spaniel. Might these experimenters have noticed the beginnings of a transformation, a metamorphosis of one creature into another?

3. Blood, Animals to Humans
(1666–1670)

When the French equivalent of the Royal Society, Louis XIV's Académie Royale des Sciences, formed in December 1666, one of its first orders of business was to recreate the blood transfusion experiments of Richard Lower.[1] The prime minister himself, Jean-Baptiste Colbert, had asked one of the Académie's founder members, Claude Perrault, to take charge of the investigation. If you've heard Perrault's name somewhere before, it's probably as the architect of the eastern facade of the Louvre Palace. Like his fellow architect Christopher Wren, though, Perrault's first interest was the human body, and he trained as a physician at Paris's Faculté de Médecine. Over three months, between December 1666 and March 1667, he teamed up with two fellow academy members, surgeon Louis Gayant and astronomer Adrien Auzout, to perform his own transfusion experiments on dogs.

But Perrault's experiments all failed in one way or another. First, he used the wrong tools. Then, when he got the tools right, the blood clotted and caked, and the three men wondered whether any blood was even getting to the dogs in the first place. To test this, they mounted two more dogs onto scales, measuring the amount of blood put in and taken out. They calculated, on one occasion, that one dog received five and a half ounces of blood, the other about six, but neither dog got away with its life. After all his experiments, he was left with nothing but piles of dead animals, so concluded that every animal's blood was made for that animal alone.

'The flesh of a dog cannot be nourished and repaired', he wrote, betraying his architectural bent, 'by the blood of another dog any more than the stone which is cut from an arch can serve either for the construction of a wall or even for another arch than that for which it was cut.'

He suspected the problem might have to do with mixing different types of blood, and that his experiments might have happier results if he could somehow make the dogs swap their blood entirely. Each would, under these circumstances, be completely emptied and refilled as one another's emittant and recipient. But this was asking too much of his equipment and skill, and why would anyone bother attempting such a thing anyway? When he wrote up his experiments, he drew on Ovid's story of Medea, just as Francis Potter had in the 1630s. He conceded that Medea had performed a useful, youth-giving transfusion, but pointed out that she also had her father-in-law drink a magical potion, which surely had something to do with the operation's success. In the absence of the fantasy potion, transfusion would remain impossible.

The truth of the matter was that, being a graduate of the faculty of medicine, Perrault was already convinced that transfusion wouldn't work. He was from the same faculty that in the fourteenth century had gone so far as to officially forbid physicians to get their hands dirty by laying them on other people's bodies. Three hundred years later, they were just as conservative: even when other medical schools around Europe had adopted Harvey's ideas, it took the physician-professors of Paris until some point in the late 1660s or early 1670s even to debate circulation. And when the evidence for circulation became irrefutable, these people still tried to preserve the ancients' prestige by insisting they had already known about circulation of blood, so it was nothing new. Back in

1666 when Perrault did his transfusion experiments, the students at his alma mater were still learning about those invisible holes in the heart and that 'wonderful net' of nerves they would never find in a human dissection.

As a former student of this faculty, Perrault inevitably had it drummed into him that Galen could not be criticized. His faith in the revered physician was so strong, in fact, that when his brother became ill with what historians think was typhoid fever, Perrault was convinced it was caused by sleeping on sheets that had been dried too near a rose bush. The 'coolness' of the roses had, he insisted, created an imbalance of humours. He started his brother's treatment, naturally enough, with bloodletting, by lancet and leech. He followed this up with a selection of enemas and chest rubs and perched a gutted pigeon on top of his head. When, after all this, his brother died, Perrault still didn't abandon Galen. He couldn't; he was a Catholic, and his Church also sanctioned these ideas.

So, when he was asked to recreate the blood-transfusion experiments, everything about it seemed to him unnatural. You were meant to take blood out, not put it in. And the noises being made across the Channel about the potential for transubstantiation would also have been objectionable to Perrault, working in Catholic Paris. Since the Académie had asked, though, it was his duty – and with the English as competition, a matter of national pride – to try. Considering his elevated professional position in the French scientific establishment, his failure to repeat Royal Society experiments and subsequent insistence that blood transfusion couldn't be done became the official line of the Parisian medical authorities.

When in January 1667 the rumours of English transfusion experiments reached the ears of Jean-Baptiste Denis, however, he was hungry to try his hand at the new procedure.

Denis was far less concerned with Galen and tradition, and with transfusion immediately saw an opportunity to make a name for himself. He'd only recently arrived in Paris from Montpellier, where he'd attended one of France's great medical schools. The faculties of Paris and Montpellier could hardly have been more different – conservative Paris barely entertained the theory of circulation, whereas forward-looking Montpellier quickly embraced it. There was also a bitter recent history between the two faculties. After Montpellier graduate Théophraste Renaudot decided to set up shop in Paris in the 1630s, the faculty charged him with practising medicine without their approval, and a prominent Parisian doctor wrote *Defence of the Faculty of Medicine of Paris*, which was an assault on Renaudot and his Montpellier-derived methods. Renaudot was driven out of business, and the faculty at Paris went so far as to formally condemn *all* doctors graduating from Montpellier. Even if Denis didn't want to go against Perrault's official ruling on blood transfusion, then, his background and training would have meant a tough start for the young doctor.

But Denis couldn't in any case have done anything straight away. He may have heard about transfusion, but he couldn't read the reports for himself. They were in English – a language he didn't understand. He wrote to the Royal Society with such desperation he was almost begging to see French translations, even offering to pay for a translation himself. But he'd have to wait. In the meantime, he offered anatomy lessons to new medical students, making his living performing the hands-on anatomy popularized by Vesalius in Italy over a hundred years earlier.

Eventually, on 31 January 1667, a full account of the English canine transfusion experiments appeared, translated into French and printed in the *Journal des sçavans*. Just as soon as he'd read about the operation, he resolved to try it out himself, starting by roping in an assistant, a well-known local surgeon, Paul Emmerez. Denis and Emmerez intended to let Denis's young medical students watch, so the two surgeons prepared them by running through the circulation process for them. With a splayed corpse rotting on the table in front of them, Denis pointed to the pathway the blood takes around the body, following its route with his finger. Being students of the medical faculty in Paris, though, their ears were closed to what they considered nonsense. They even had to suppress their laughter as Denis pointed to the digestive system and ran his finger up to the heart.

He would have gone on to say, if his students hadn't descended into hysterics, that circulation was nothing but the constant transfusion of blood from part to part. Circulation had convinced Denis that transfusion was not only possible, it was natural. He used pregnancy as an example of constant transfusion between two bodies, mother and baby, who are physically tethered as 'one and the same Body and Substance'. The foetus is nourished by transfusion, which, as Denis put it, 'vivifies' and 'encreases all the parts'.[2] Trying to convince a Parisian student of even the most fundamental aspects of Harvey's theory was pointless, however, so at that very early stage Denis and Emmerez made their preparations behind closed doors.

They chose their next audience more carefully. In front of a small hand-picked selection of dignitaries, Denis and Emmerez tied up their first dogs, head to tail, and performed their transfusion following Lower's method, connecting the two circulatory systems with a couple of tubes. But going further than Lower, the two French surgeons nursed *both* dogs back to health. On 8 March 1667, they went further still and set up a transfusion between three dogs. Dog 1 was bled into dog 2, who was bled into dog 3, who was bled into dog 1. All three dogs survived this ordeal, too.

Only a day later, Denis wrote a report for the *Journal des sçavans* – the publication that had reported on Lower's experiments in England – and announced that he was planning to perform the transplant experiment for the public, on the banks of the Seine at 2 p.m. on Saturday, 12 March. 'So you can see what changes transfusion can produce,' Denis wrote, 'we will transfer the blood of a young and healthy dog into the veins of an old and mangy one.' For the site of his demonstration, Denis had chosen the Pont Neuf – as much a marketplace as a bridge, with street theatre and tooth pulling, pickpockets and glass-eye salesmen. And, for one day only, at the foot of this landmark, Denis would perform a live blood transfusion. A good crowd had gathered, and once again Denis and Emmerez strapped down a young dog and secured an old dog next to it. Following Lower's procedure, the two dogs once more survived, this time to the cheers of a crowd. Denis became a minor celebrity that day, and though still only surviving on proceeds from anatomy lessons, it wouldn't be long before he could ramp up his experiments.

Anonymized in Denis's audience at the foot of the Pont Neuf was a sixty-seven-year-old aristocrat, Henri-Louis de Montmor.[3] The Montmor family had been a prominent and well-connected part of Parisian society for two centuries. Montmor's father was the Master of Requests (a high-level legal-administrative appointment) for King Henri IV, and oversaw the war treasury, a position to which his son had succeeded him by the age of thirty-two. Montmor was once a big deal in Parisian scientific circles, but at the time of Denis's demonstration had recently suffered a spectacular fall. Certain rich Parisian men at the time telegraphed both their wealth and supposed intelligence by buying and showing off scientific curiosities such as sundials, microscopes and clocks. In the Marais, the district in which Montmor lived, efforts at social manoeuvring became so ridiculous amongst the residents that telescopes protruded from roofs, each man wanting a bigger and more powerful eyepiece than his neighbour. These lenses – 'deadly weapons from the roofs of peaceful citizens', as one historian put it – became the centrepieces of so-called 'observation parties', where the owner's friends would take it in turns to sit at the giant lens and gawp at Venus or the moon. In some exceptional cases, Montmor's included, the owners of these peculiar houses bankrolled their own learned 'societies', effectively adding clever men to their collections of scientific curios. Montmor had his own Académie Montmor, which he had set up in 1653, but it had recently collapsed.

In its heyday, the aristocrat would invite the greatest scientific minds to dine and pontificate at his expense. He'd give them space, instruments and access to his sprawling library. Before their meetings they'd tuck into elaborate dinners that included delicacies shipped from all corners of the New World, washed down with wine from his own vineyard. He would go to great lengths to woo the minds he thought would bring him the most prestige, and even the great philosopher René Descartes dined at his table. Montmor found another star to court in the Dutch astronomer Christiaan Huygens (also famous for inventing the pendulum clock). It was in Montmor's great library, in fact, that Huygens reported his greatest discovery – the rings surrounding Saturn, the appearance of which had stumped Galileo (whose own telescope happened to stand only feet away in Montmor's window). By extension, Huygens made Montmor a grand figure in the scientific community in Paris. Montmor truly had the biggest telescope on the block.

Montmor's trouble started when the secretary of Académie Montmor, Samuel de Sorbière, saw an opportunity for his own advancement. Sorbière was an admirer of the English philosopher Thomas Hobbes, who felt that human beings were better off under authoritarian government. Without strong structures to organize them, he thought, humankind would never achieve anything. There would be no industry, no art, no science and no society as people pressed individual claims to whatever they liked. The 'life of man' under such a system – or rather lack of system – would, he wrote, be 'solitary, poor, nasty, brutish, and short'. Sorbière approved of this sentiment and created structures in Montmor's society to respond solely to Montmor's whims, as the figure of absolute authority.

Throughout his time as secretary of Montmor's society, Sorbière naturally kept himself in the loop when it came to royal affairs. King Louis XIV had just chosen his new prime minister, Jean-Baptiste Colbert, and dispensed with one toadying pretender by locking him up. Though young, the king was decisive, and this promise of strong authority impressed Sorbière. He decided to petition the new prime minister, asking him to fund a national scientific endeavour similar to the Royal Society in England.

One evening, Sorbière delivered an impassioned speech to Montmor's entire assembly. First, he thanked Montmor for his service to science. 'We can only hope that he will continue to show his commitment to his glory and for the public utility by allowing the Academy to pass into the hands of the sovereign.' Science was important to the nation, he said, and private scientific concerns like Montmor's must be consolidated for the good of France. Until science became a national

concern, with the kind of funding only a nation could provide, 'our Medicine will be blind, and our Sciences will teach
us with certainty only that there is an infinity of things about
which we know nothing'. Montmor listened to every treach-
erous word. And with snake-like cunning, Sorbière sent a
copy of his speech to the Palace, along with a letter to the
prime minister. Though Sorbière insisted he had nothing to
gain from sharing his speech, the prime minister saw through
his manoeuvring. But he supported the formation of a royal
academy of science anyway after witnessing a solar eclipse
and comet shower – the same comet shower that many
thought foretold the Plague and Great Fire of London. It
was, he realized, in the national interest to understand, rather
than fear, nature and the movement of the stars.

The new Académie Royale des Sciences was formed and
led by an even more illustrious figure than Montmor – the
Sun King himself, Louis XIV, whose gravitational pull
seemed to attract luminaries from all Paris's private societies.
Montmor's private academy was bled of its savants as even
Huygens abandoned the humiliated aristocrat for the stipend
and rooms in the king's library. The reluctant transfusionist
Claude Perrault, who knew the prime minister personally,
joined the Académie from the society of Montmor's rival,
Melchisédech Thiévenot. Worse still, the prime minister had
asked one of Montmor's friends for a list of those worthy of
royal recognition, and Montmor's name wasn't on it.

When the ageing nobleman watched Denis and Emmerez
confidently coupling up two dogs on the banks of the Seine,
Montmor must have seen a way to reverse his social fortunes.
Maybe he even felt Denis offered him a route to revenge.
Whatever went through his mind, it was thanks to the injured
fortunes of this bitter old man that Denis gained a sponsor,

one who would tie his own reputation to the success of his blood-transfusion efforts. So, in spite of official condemnation from the Académie Royale des Sciences, Denis now had the means to act in direct opposition to Perrault's ruling. And he had an insanely rich supporter with the political appetite to encourage him.

Having no doubt read Boyle's sixteen directions for transfusion, Denis started a new series of experiments, setting up in Montmor's private garden in April 1667. Montmor himself stood by to watch as his ostler heaved a terrified calf onto a blood stained table, and next to it a dog. For the first time ever, Denis and Emmerez made the blood of the young cow flow through their network of tubes and into the body of the dog. He did this three times and reported that not only did all the animals survive, they didn't even lose their appetites. Even the weakest one, who retreated and cowered after its transfusion, eventually 'showed a surprising vigour'.[4] Over the days and weeks, Denis continued experimenting on more animals, transfusing three sheep into three dogs, more cows into dogs, and a horse into four goats.

Though Denis was an outlier in France, he was by no means the only transfusionist operating in Europe. Within a month of Denis's experiments, Edmund King reported similar experiments he'd performed in England. He found transfusing a calf's blood into a sheep made it 'very strong and lusty'. Thomas Coxe had also been conducting the young-and-healthy-into-old-and-mangy kind of transfusion. Within a fortnight, he found, he'd cured a mangy dog. The Italians were also getting into transfusion. In April, Giovanni Cassini transfused sheep, and in May dogs, cows, goats and horses. Paolo Manfredi and Guglielmo Riva made their own experiments, as did Ippolito Magnani, who also made his own glass transfusion tubes, which he found made the blood flow much more easily. For this short time in April and May 1667, it seemed Denis had plenty of competition. But he had plans to move it to the next level.

The World's First Xeno-Transfusions

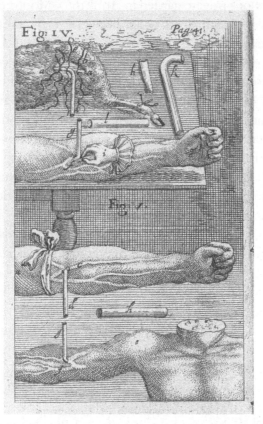

Figure 16 Image from a German textbook depicting a transfusion between animals and humans, 1667.

One day in the middle of June 1667, Denis was called to the bedside of a teenage boy who'd been thrown into disarray by a violent fever. Over the preceding two months, physicians had bled the boy twenty times to 'asswage the excessive heat' and he'd lost his energy, memory and wits. When Denis and Emmerez came to see him on 15 June 1667, he was looking pasty and weak from loss of blood. As the two doctors punctured the boy's skin, they reported, nothing but a thick, black ooze of blood seeped out. Denis took Emmerez to one side and explained that there wasn't enough blood in this lad's body for it to be circulating at all. It must be sitting stagnant in pools, unable to deliver its life- and energy-giving properties. Even as they bled their patients dry, doctors had always known that blood roughly equated to life. Galenic doctors wrote about 'innate spirit' carried through the body, which was vital to existence in general, and it was an explanation as to why living bodies are warm – they have an 'innate heat' and 'primitive moisture'. The medieval guidelines on phlebotomy added that elderly people should not be bled because they couldn't afford to lose what little life remained in their bodies. The seventeenth-century physician Joseph Glanvill called bloodletting the 'grand inconvenience' for this very reason. The boy at Denis's side clearly needed more blood not less, so they sent someone to find a suitable donor.

They returned, naturally enough, with a bleating lamb. We eat animals and drink their milk and blood, after all, so it was logical to suppose we could assimilate their blood directly. But it was really 'pure' blood the two transfusionists were after. They wanted to give the patient the strength that came with blood coursing around his body, but didn't want to pass on an armful of the stuff that was corrupt. Human blood, of course, would have been the most corrupt, and therefore least desirable option. People swear too much, have sex when they're not supposed to and are otherwise prone to 'debauchery', Denis said, and have 'irregular' eating and drinking habits. All this affects the quality of their blood. Even children sucked 'corruption together with their nourishment' in a debauched mother's milk. But animals, especially the lambs of God, are innocent, so what blood could be purer? And what's more, since we can tell how an animal was fed by just tasting its meat, eggs or milk, it must be possible to distinguish between different qualities of blood and even, theoretically, to design blood for a specific transfusion. Denis took some steps in this direction, in fact, proposing that it would be 'expedient', as he put it, to prepare the emittant animal by feeding it an appropriate diet in the days running up to the operation.

He may have been on the wrong track, but this way of thinking makes Denis one of the most inventive, brilliant minds I've ever come across. Harvey gave us a partly mechanical body; Denis, however, treated the old humoral system as if it, too, was mechanical. When you put aside the more 'magical' or illogical dimensions of humoralism, such as its reliance on astronomy, it becomes a matter of managing fluids. To correct someone's temperament, the amount of corrupt blood had to be reduced. But it was impossible to isolate corrupt blood, and bleed that alone, because blood gushed in a single stream. The usual bloodletting treatment would lower the overall amount of blood, but this would sometimes be too much. If you could fill up a patient with pure – or, better still, specially designed – animal blood, you could cut down the level of corrupt blood to whatever you liked and increase the overall amount of blood to a safe level. Transfusion would in this way add a new lever to the humoral machine, making a mechanical system of something that was never anything of the kind. This is surely genius.

With the conviction that a lamb's blood would naturally be the purest of them all, Denis acted in direct opposition to Perrault. He and Emmerez tied down the lamb and inserted a tube into an artery in its neck – the carotid artery to catch the blood on its way from the lamb's heart to its brain. Next, it was the boy's turn to have a tube inserted. They chose a vein in his arm. In the next moment, they brought the two tubes together. And they started to count. They left the two bodies connected until they judged enough lamb blood had entered the boy to restore his 'vital heat' and dilute his fever. When the two transfusionists guessed he'd had enough, they pulled apart their temporary connection. The boy said he felt a 'great heat' along his arm as the new blood entered his body.

The boy was put to bed, where he dropped off to sleep.

When he awoke he was 'cheerful enough'. He then ate for the rest of the day 'with much more liveliness than ordinary'. 'Now', wrote Denis, 'he executes nimbly whatever is appointed him, and he hath no longer that slowness of spirit nor grows fat visibly.' The first animal–human blood transfusion was a great success. Contrary to what Richard Lower's findings suggested might happen, it even seemed to make the recipient a bit more lamb-like.

Soon after, Denis and Emmerez repeated the operation on a forty-five-year-old butcher. His transfusion was a pure experiment. There was nothing wrong with him, but Denis and Emmerez wanted to make some observations so paid him to take in the lamb's blood and let them watch how he responded. The two transfusionists gave him one transfusion of ten ounces and two more doses of twenty. Like the

boy before him, he became more active and cheerful afterwards, but seemed otherwise unaffected by the transfusions.
Denis wanted him to stay awhile so he could compare his
behaviour with that of the lad they'd transfused earlier. Even
though he was being paid, the butcher refused to comply.
Denis found him in the pub later, wine glass in hand. He'd in
the meantime put his butchery skills to good use and jointed
and eaten his donor. As Denis vented his anger at his irre-
sponsible research subject, he was at least able to see that the
butcher was well and energetic.

Almost immediately, Denis wrote up his experiment in a
letter to his sponsor, Montmor, which he also had printed
and distributed around Paris and sent to England. Denis
wanted to be known as the first person to conduct animal-
to-human blood transfusions. And this was true. But he
neglected to acknowledge any of the English experimenters
who had preceded him. Before blowing your own trumpet,
the convention in scientific communication was to acknowledge your influences, and Denis didn't even mention William
Harvey.

Not only did he paper over his English predecessors, he
claimed they had played no part at all. In Denis's letter, we
learn about a Benedictine monk, Dom Robert Desgabets,
who apparently first proposed blood transfusion in Montmor's
academy back in 1658 – earlier than Lower's experiments.
Desgabets had suggested collecting blood in a small leather
bag and pouring it into the body through a silver pipe with a
funnel on top. Though no one ever tried this method, Denis
wrote, it was proof that blood transfusion was a French
invention. The historian Holly Tucker – who has closely
studied the dealings of Montmor's academy – found no
mention of this mysterious Benedictine monk in any of the

academy's papers, other than Denis's own. In 1658 the Montmor scientists weren't even particularly interested in medicine – this was the time of Huygens's studies of Saturn and the astronomical observation parties with the giant telescopes. And Denis would have been twenty-two at the time, still at medical school in Montpellier, so even if this wasn't a fabrication, he would have lived too far away and cut too insignificant a figure to have been invited to Montmor's meeting.[5]

When Denis's letter reached England, it was received with plenty of hostility. One doctor, Timothy Clarke, later responded with a letter going through the history of transfusion in detail, from Francis Potter right through the creation of ivory pipes and quills twenty years later, to his own work with Christopher Wren, where they injected 'waters, various kinds of beer, milk and whey, broths, wines, alcohol, and the blood of different animals'. Finishing with his account of Richard Lower's ground-breaking transfusions, he concluded that 'the honour for this invention – if it deserves any – should be awarded to the English rather than the French'.[6] Denis was so far out of line that even Louis XIV's secretary wrote to the Royal Society, telling them how dishonourable Denis's behaviour was. But although the claims surrounding the French origins of his animal–human experiments were dubious, Denis had still, irrefutably, been the first to conduct transfusions on humans.

With wounded English pride, Edmund King wrote that he and Richard Lower had been wanting for six months to try an animal–human transfusion, but had been waiting for 'the removal of some considerations of a Moral Nature'. Some of their fellow Royal Society members had objected to transfusion in the past, but when the society's German-born secretary, Henry Oldenburg, suggested that transfusion 'be prosecuted' safely on human beings, the motion was supported with enthusiasm. The Royal Society hurriedly made Lower into a fellow – which, surprisingly, he hadn't been until this point – and found him and King rooms overlooking the Thames. These would serve as their laboratory.

Later that autumn, ex-Queen Christina of Sweden called on Denis and Emmerez in Paris. She wanted to know if they'd perform a blood transfusion for her former adviser, Baron Bond.[7] The Parisian physician Pierre Bourdelot had previously written to Christina, a former patient of his, and piqued her interest in blood transfusion. She wouldn't want to try it herself, she wrote back to tell him, in case she turned into a sheep, but on second thoughts she wouldn't mind metamorphosing into a 'female lion so that no one could devour me'. Or maybe she'd try the blood of a German, because they're 'less like a human being than is any other animal I know'. But when she heard Bond had been taken seriously ill in Paris, she sent for Denis and Emmerez.

The Bond who lay there to greet them was almost unconscious, and Denis and Emmerez were nervous about transfusing him. He was already very ill, probably close to death. It looked to them like a diseased liver and spleen. But after a night's rest, Denis and Emmerez concluded that transfusion might be his only hope, and returned with a calf. The pair of transfusionists hooked up the two creatures with their silver tubes, as usual, and the blood started to flow. With countless experiments on dogs and two human patients under their belts, Denis and Emmerez were getting better at transfusion. Pulling the tube away, they left Bond to sleep.

He woke revived enough to drink some broth, but soon started to fade. So, they repeated the transfusion, working as quickly as possible. Denis and Emmerez wouldn't have known that platelets would naturally stick to the side of their silver tube if they took too long to make the transfusion. This was probably what was happening all along. Obstructing the flow of blood would have meant their patients got little or no blood inside them after all. Some would have made it through – and a human body can deal with a small amount of animal blood with only relatively mild symptoms – enough to provoke a fever and fatigue, but not enough to kill. Denis was clearly getting better, quicker, at physically getting the blood out of one body and into another because Bond died from his new calf blood shortly after a second transfusion.

Bond had been bled, of course, before the two transfusionists arrived, and Denis was convinced things would have worked out differently had they been called beforehand. They'd even made the physicians who'd bled him admit they were wrong to do so before permitting the transfusion. And Denis still proclaimed the operation a success. His patient might have died, but this was because he was too ill, and transfusion couldn't be expected to cure every disease at all stages.

It seems news of Bond's treatment and death never reached the Royal Society, who were busy hunting for a patient for Lower and King to experiment on at their new laboratory beside the Thames. At one of their next meetings, the venerable voice of George Ent – friend of the late William Harvey and founding member of Charles Scarburgh's group – spoke up. The transfusionists should, he proposed, try transfusing blood to 'some mad person in the hospital of Bethlem'. In the early seventeenth century, some still considered madness to be caused by divine or demonic possession and witchcraft. Drilling a hole in the head would supposedly let out the demons, and now and then a doctor would convince himself there was a small 'stone' lodged in his patient's head, and would rummage around to find it. According to Robert Burton's 1628 *Anatomy of Melancholy*, though, stones had nothing to do with madness, which was instead caused by 'idleness, solitariness, overmuch study, passions, perturbations, discontents, cares, miseries, vehement desires, ambitions, etc.'. Amongst the usual herbal cures, diet and even music therapy, Burton recommended the ubiquitous bloodletting treatment be applied to the forehead to draw the blood away from the brain and cool it. The 'cooling effects' of blood transfusion, agreed Lower and his fellow transfusion experimenters, might work as a treatment for madness. As it happened, Thomas Allen – the director of the mental asylum – wouldn't consent to their pressing his lunatics into service for transfusion experiments, and when they knocked at his door in the hope they could convince him in person, he sent them on their way.

Having been turned away from Bedlam, Lower and King had to find their own lunatic. When they reported back to the Royal Society, another voice from the recent past had an idea. This time it was John Wilkins. He told the assembly that, at church on Sunday, sitting at a nearby pew had been an eccentric man, or maybe he was mildly insane, about thirty-two years old. Henry Oldenburg chipped in to describe him as 'very freakish and extravagant', but this man had studied Theology at Cambridge and, the fellows reasoned, could even speak intelligently about how the blood affected him. His name was Arthur Coga, and he agreed to be their guinea pig on condition that he could relate his experiences in Latin – his preferred tongue.

On 23 November 1667 Lower and King's laboratory was so full of Royal Society members, MPs and eminent doctors they had to push their way through the throng to get to their patient.[8] Crammed in front of a crowd all jostling to get a good view, the surgeons opened a lamb's artery and let it bleed into a cup, timing its stream. As they were calculating the flow rate – which was twelve ounces of blood per minute – Coga dipped a knife into the dish and brought it up to his lips, pronouncing the blood to be 'of good relish' as he held his arm out to the doctors. Lower and King made their incision into a vein in Coga's arm, and immediately plugged it. They did the same with the wound in the bleeding lamb and went to connect the silver tubes and hollow quills together, constructing a corridor for the blood to flow through. As they unstoppered the two wounds, the lamb's blood started to make its way through their apparatus and into the arm of Coga, who told the assembled crowd that he couldn't feel the same 'heat' Denis's patients reportedly felt. The lamb blood flowed straight into Coga's veins for two minutes.

When he'd had enough, King pulled the pipe out and the ovine blood continued to trickle out onto the laboratory floor. The spectators all had questions, and the talkative research subject was keen to answer them. They plied Coga with wine and tobacco as King sewed up his arm. He told the crowd that he was very happy to have lamb's blood circulating his body because of its symbolic association – 'Christ is the Lamb of God', he said (in Latin). With his finger on Coga's pulse, King announced that it was 'stronger and fuller' than before the operation, and the crowd cheered.

After his transfusion, Coga toddled off pretty much un-affected and Lower and King tipped the donor's carcass and its giblets into the river. From home, Coga reported that he had a good appetite, and produced the usual 'three or four stools'.

But later his condition deteriorated, and he started to sweat uncontrollably. When Wilkins and Oldenburg – perhaps the two Royal Society members who knew him best – went to visit him in the morning, he was exhausted. But he was no longer behaving in that 'freakish and extravagant' manner.

Feeling like a new man, Coga came back for more on 12 December, having eight ounces of his own blood taken out and fourteen of sheep put in. The diarist Samuel Pepys was in the audience, and wrote that, though he spoke well, Coga still seemed 'cracked a little in his head'. And some voices from the crowd heckled the two transfusionists. They didn't believe the blood was getting into Coga and wanted subjects to be weighed before and after.

The Royal Society planned another transfusion for Coga, which is something they might have tried had they not received a letter from someone called Agnus Coga. The mysterious correspondent complained that Arthur had sold his clothes and was now poor because he'd started to turn into a sheep, and no one would employ such a creature. The letter went on to say that he would take part in a third experiment only if they promised to complete the metamorphosis. It's not clear who was writing under the moniker 'Agnus Coga', 'Coga the Lamb'. Whoever wrote it, Arthur Coga was never seen again.

The scientific and medical communities beyond the Royal Society had surprisingly little to say about transfusion. The English physician Henry Stubbe, writing in 1670, worried that one creature's blood would be incompatible with another's, even if they were of the same species, as different kinds of blood coagulated at different points.[9] He went so far as to claim that it was possible to taste the difference between male and female blood. The ill effects of transfusion would be

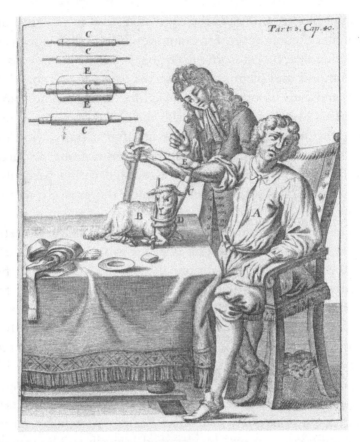

Figure 17 Transfusion of lamb's blood to human, 1705.

'absolutely past remedy', he said, because blood could not be taken back out. George Acton, another English doctor, felt that blood of all kinds was full of 'vital spirit' and 'volatile salt', so any creature that has blood can't be too dissimilar. It should in theory be possible for blood to be 'easily transmuted and assimilated', which would fortify the patient and help him overcome his disease. Acton even offered a list of animal bloods and gave their potential uses in transfusion. Ass blood cures fever, for example, while a colt's cures yellow jaundice. Blood from a male goat cures the lung diseases pneumonia and pleurisy. Dysentery? Ox blood will sort that out, and cat's blood should be used for falling sickness and herpes. Gout can be treated with the blood of a male deer, and bladder stones should clear up after a transfusion of fox's blood. Each animal's 'vital spirit' was not only a source of life itself, but also a quality associated with a particular creature. It was a matter of matching the creature to the disease.[10]

Despite a smattering of scientists taking transfusion seriously, there is a good deal of evidence to suggest that much of the population thought transfusion was a joke, and the suggestion that anyone might actually be transformed by animal blood was worth a good laugh. Members of the Royal Society had form in pursuing seemingly pointless goals that were easily satirized. Wren's mentor, John Wilkins, would, for example, invent a so-called 'universal language' he thought might replace Latin. Unlike a natural language, which was organic and unpredictable, Wilkins's universal language was carefully structured. Each word would refer to a specific concept and be classified logically.[11] The satirist Jonathan Swift would later parody Wilkins's language in *Gulliver's Travels*, when the academy of Lagado proposed a universally understood language of their own, replacing words with objects people would carry around in sacks.[12]

Long before *Gulliver's Travels*, in 1676, a new play came out ridiculing the Royal Society: *The Virtuoso*, by Thomas Shadwell.[13] It, too, featured a transfusionist, Sir Nicholas Grimcrack (a play on 'gimcrack', a cheap and garish trinket). He was the virtuoso – another name for experimenters like

Lower, Boyle and Wren – and featured alongside his colleagues Sir Formal Trifle and Old Snarl. These characters dabbled in pointless experiments, mostly to do with measuring air – a real-life preoccupation of the early Royal Society, and something that Pepys and even Charles II had poked fun at as inherently stupid. The king, in fact, made it to one of Shadwell's first performances of the play, and saw Sir Nicholas bragging about something even sillier than measuring air – transfusing sixty-four ounces of blood from one sheep into a madman. The sheep died, but the madman was still alive, though he suffered a bit at first as their bloodstreams merged. Then all of a sudden, he let out a bleat. And he started chewing the cud, grew wool and sprouted a Northamptonshire sheep's tail out of his 'humane fundament'. Sir Nicholas concludes that he must make an entire flock of sheep using blood transfusion, turn the wool into clothes and make his fortune.

Back in Paris, Denis had deadly serious detractors and they were in no mood to laugh. While the inventive young transfusionist was busy spreading the word about his operations in late 1667, another Parisian physician called Pierre-Martin de la Martinière received a divine command to stop him and warn the world of the menace materializing on the horizon.[14] No sooner had he put his head on his pillow and drifted off to sleep than he saw Apollo standing in his bedroom, bow in one hand, lyre in the other. The Goddess of Truth appeared, too, and washed Martinière's eyes 'so', Apollo told him, 'you can see what I want to show you'. With that, Apollo commanded Martinière to 'spread the message to the rest of the human race', as the goddess snatched back the bed curtains to reveal a precipice below.

Martinière craned his neck over the side of his bed and

felt death fill his nostrils as he squinted to bring into focus the scene below. A group of natural philosophers were looking for the secret of immortality and fancied they found it in the blood. One grabbed a helpless animal – Martinière was not specific about the species – and sliced off its tail. As it fell to the floor, the philosopher stuffed a syringe where the tail used to be and forced milk into its body, echoing what Richard Lower had done back in real-life England. He tried to stuff so much milk into the creature, it oozed out of its eye sockets, nostrils and ears. As if channelling the Oxford experiments, the dream-philosopher proclaimed: 'those who can no longer eat can now introduce food into their veins'.

The others nodded their approval, and each grabbed a pair of animals for a transfusion party. They transfused lion's blood into a lamb, lamb's blood into a wolf. One of the philosophers upped the ante by sticking his bloodied lancet into one of his colleagues and bled him dry. Martinière watched, wide-eyed, gripping his blankets as the scene played out below his bed, while the philosophers coupled their colleague's body to a cow and let the blood flow from beast to man. As the bovine transfusion came to an end, the recipient's arms and legs slowly morphed into hooves, and his human head swelled and bulged. This wasn't right, but it was too late. As the philosopher's eyes grew huge and brown to complete his transformation, his colleagues panicked and the curtain came down around Martinière's bed, his dream over.

That morning Martinière awoke with a start, but it was really just the beginning of his nightmare. His servant pushed open the door, bringing the morning light in with him, and three letters. The first was a copy of the one Denis wrote for Montmor, detailing his successful transfusions between dogs, other animals and, finally, the two human transfusions involving the young boy and the butcher. Perhaps his sense of foreboding was heightened by the previous night's dream, but this letter convinced Martinière that the transfusionist had done nothing but create a market for blood. Foreshadowing the dark days of eighteenth-century transplants, he imagined future merchants brokering deals for the rich to buy the blood of the poor, and children being offered up in medical sacrifice. They'd be whipped, he thought, to bring blood to the surface of their tiny bodies, and drained of every drop of liquid, all in the hope their precious fluid would cure the terrible diseases suffered by the wealthy. 'Men will cut one another's throats', he said, 'to preserve their life.' They would bathe in blood if they thought it would cure them of something. Blood transfusion, he thought, was just one step removed from cannibalism.

He'd already seen similarly despicable behaviour in Egypt, where he'd formed this poor opinion of his fellow humans. Though he was now a physician in the court of Louis XIV, he'd taken some interesting turns to get there. He'd run away from home when he was nine and tagged along with a barber surgeon, learning his trade in a military encampment near Geneva. When he was twelve, the Spanish captured his regiment and the young surgeon-to-be talked his way onto a Portuguese ship bound for the Barbary Coast. Pirates boarded the ship and its surgeon died in the conflict. When the pirates interrogated the remaining crew, Martinière declared himself to be the surgeon, took over his dead colleague's tools and inherited his trade in the service of the pirates.

While replenishing his medicine chest one day in an Egyptian apothecary, Martinière happened to see dried-up and flaking human bodies piled one on top of the other. These were mummies stacked for export to the European market, where some of the most respected doctors would prescribe them. They thought that eating the skin of a mummy – either gnawing on it directly or ingesting it as fine grains – was the cure for all kinds of diseases. Alongside these withered specimens, a man was busy tapping into the head and chest of a newly dead body. Martinière watched as the man replaced the fresh internal organs with a sticky black liquid and wrapped the body up, then putting it beside the others to dry out. Taking a sprinkle of Egyptian mummy in the morning became a treatment so sought after in Europe that the supply of real mummies started to run low, and the exporters turned to smallpox, plague and leprosy victims. It was the remains of *these* bodies the man was processing into medicine. As Martinière watched the ship being loaded with chunks of fresh mummy, the sight marked him for ever. Not long after, he was liberated by the Knights of Malta. He was still only sixteen, but he'd lost whatever taste for piracy he might have had.

The former pirate then worked for a spell as an assistant to an alchemist, keeping the fire going as his employer heated various chemicals and materials in his search for eternal life. 'After having puffed three days and three nights with someone without accomplishing anything but wasting our time, our fuel and all of our lead, I took a bat and smashed all of the furnaces, kettles, alembics and cauldrons,' he later wrote. And he swore he would never again 'pursue the mad search for the so-called Philosopher's Stone'.

He then worked in a Roman hospital before making his way back to Rouen, where he went to medical school and officially became a physician. By the mid-to-late 1660s

Martinière had reinvented himself and was living a life completely transformed as a physician in Paris. But he never forgot the sight of those newly created mummies being shipped back to Europe for fellow humans to eat, and it came back to him when he read Denis's letter. It gets slightly easier to believe human beings would bay for one another's blood if you've already seen bodies being prepared for eating.

If the first letter reminded him a little too much of the previous night's nightmare, the second letter he opened that day made things worse. It, too, was about blood transfusion and was from a Parisian doctor called Guillaume Lamy. Lamy was one of Denis's staunchest critics, in fact, and had reams of objections to his practices, all resonating with what Martinière thought himself. It's all very well transplanting calmness, meekness or other virtuous qualities, but maybe laziness or stupidity could also be transferred, he thought. In letters recently translated by Holly Tucker, he explained how blood has 'particles' inside it, giving its owner a specific character. A cow's particles makes a cow stupid, so if you transfuse a cow's blood, you'll transfuse bovine dullness along with it. Transferring blood also transferred the soul, he thought, so although the Protestant English might laugh at the idea, for Lamy, a recipient of animal blood would literally start to turn into the 'inferior animal'. An ox's blood, he wrote, couldn't nourish a man, and a sheep's blood would transfer the woolly part of the animal's soul, so the recipient would grow a fleece. As a point of principle, he felt doctors should recognize that interfering with the blood interfered with the identity, the self, essence, nature, soul. They should take care 'not to wound the soul, by curing the diseases of the body'. All people are individuals, Lamy thought, and this is due to them all having different blood. If people could be made stupid, sprout wool or grow hooves, they would also lose their humanity.

The monsters had leapt out of the poetry, and now threatened to invade real life. The barriers between one person and another, between humans and animals even, had just been dissolved by an upstart doctor from Montpellier. The world had so far been lucky that a man's death was the worst thing to happen.

And if by some miracle he was wrong, and transfusing animal blood turned out to be effective, Lamy complained, there wouldn't be enough animals in the world to deal with all the sick. But what truly terrified Lamy was the possibility of the boundaries between bodies and souls collapsing and different lives running up against one another, mixing and mingling; the creation of monsters as in Ovid's terrifying stories. For Lamy the soul was *part of* the body, and the body *part of* the soul, with the blood the 'harmonious link', as he put it, between the two. Martinière, on the same page as Lamy, thought 'to allow foreign blood to enter one's veins is to bring about a blood bath', to 'attract the ire of God'.

The third letter – which was actually a defence of Denis, directly refuting Lamy's criticism – did nothing to ameliorate Martinière's attitude towards transfusion. For Martinière, the matter was decided. He'd already been convinced of the human race's capacity for evil in the brief time he was a pirate surgeon. And over the next few nights Martinière was visited by more dreams where he was pitted in mortal combat against the various monsters created by blood transfusion. He saw and fought a chimera with the head of a lion, tail of a dragon and stomach of a goat. He went to slash at the monster, but some 'learned men' threatened him into submission.

Athena arrived next, brandishing a javelin, and thrashed the monster with a club. On another night, Martinière dreamed of Medea. 'She looked at me with angry eyes', Martinière later wrote, and told him 'if my charms are not strong enough to convince you to give up your resolve to abolish transfusion, I will rip you apart as I did my brother and the children that I had with Jason'. Then Martinière lashed out against Medea, calling her a 'deadly witch', vowing to do everything he could to stop her transfusionist message.

Where blood transfusionists had presented Medea as a kind of mythical precedent, they recollected only so much of her story – up to the rejuvenation of Jason's father. Martinière remembered the darker second half, where Medea turned murderous, tricking Pelias's daughters into slitting their own father's throat, and then taking flight in her magical chariot. During her journey across the known world, looking down on a planet ravaged by unnatural, sinister transformations, she saw the lake where Cygnus turned into a swan after jumping off a cliff. Thinking her son dead, his mother wept so heavily she metamorphosed into Lake Hyrie. She looked to the left and saw the fields of Calavera, Leto's island, whose king and his wife transformed into birds. She looked to the right and, in the distance, saw Cephissus, lamenting the fate of his grandson who had been changed by Apollo into a bloated seal.[15] This was the true danger, Martinière thought, of letting blood transfusionists have their way.

Martinière's fears about transfusion were singular, but nevertheless resonated with a more general sense of anxiety about transmutation in France. While an acceptable subject for a Protestant to ponder, bodily transformation or transubstantiation was blasphemy for Catholics. And, since

Denis was imitating the English – traditional enemies of the French – pursuing transfusion might also be considered treasonous. Rallying around all their imagined and real objections to Denis and transfusion, a dedicated group of physicians began to organize themselves around Martinière and Lamy, a group who would stop at nothing to disrupt Denis's most dangerous occupation.

On 19 December 1667, just a week after Lower and King succeeded in transforming Arthur into Agnus Coga, Denis was picked up in Montmor's carriage and rolled into his city estate. A valet conducted him to the grand room with vaulted ceiling. There, around a gigantic stone fireplace, were gathered a special group of guests, including Pierre Bourdelot (the physician who wrote to Christina, the former queen of Sweden, and in the times before the Académie Royale des Sciences, once a convenor of his own Académie Bourdelot) and Louis de Buade de Frontenac (Montmor's brother-in-law, a courtier who would in 1672 become Governor General of New France, the French colonies in Canada). Montmor himself greeted the young doctor. There were two tables in the centre of the room. Emmerez was already arranging instruments on one, while Montmor's ostler helped a butcher – perhaps even the same butcher Denis had operated on earlier in the year – lift a calf onto another. The calf writhed, and the two men struggled to restrain the pathetic creature, finally punching it into submission. Its terrified noise was soon drowned out by an equally terrified man, restrained and dragged into the room by Montmor's guards. The butcher and stableman finished securing the calf and rushed to help the guards rope the man into an adjacent chair, as Montmor and his assembly watched.

The man's name was Antoine Mauroy.[16] He was naked,

except for a few rags tied loosely around his body. He'd been gallivanting around in the mud on the banks of the Seine when Montmor's footmen picked him up. Mauroy had once been respectable. He had been the Marquise de Sévigné's valet but had gradually descended into insanity. He'd fallen for a woman of superior birth, who ended up marrying another higher-class man, leaving poor Mauroy to a bitterness that was too much for him. The Sévigné household had dismissed Mauroy about four years previously, in 1663, because he'd tried to set the house on fire. Receiving the news, he tore his uniform from his body and ran out into the streets naked, and had since been found, on occasion, roaming around Paris unclothed and setting fire to things. Soon after, he married a local woman, Perrine, who believed his family when they told her his insanity had passed. But he beat her. Still, she went out into the streets looking for him whenever he went missing, leading him home and getting friends to help tie him down to stop him hurting himself or anyone else. One story goes that cavalry guards were patrolling the Marais and trotted their horses over to an archway to feed on some hay lying there. But the first horse's nose butted a naked Mauroy, who was using the hay as his bed. Mauroy leapt up, screamed and yanked the horse's tail, causing it to bolt. Now Mauroy was tied up in Montmor's library. The old aristocrat hoped Denis and Emmerez could cure him. Perrine wasn't present. She was panicking her way around Paris looking for her lost husband.

Where old-school physicians might have kept their distance, manual work being beneath them, Denis and Emmerez went right up to Mauroy. To treat the obvious madness, local barber surgeons had already bled him eighteen times to no avail. They'd also given him potions and a herbal bath, but his condition was the same as ever. They looked and prodded their way around his body for signs of disease. There was none. They were reassured that, unlike their last patient, he was physically fit. It was just his blood, his personality, his soul that was disordered. On this occasion, it made sense to give Mauroy some new blood 'to improve his character'.

Emmerez drew ten ounces of Mauroy's blood, to make room for the calf's. Jostled by the crowd gathered in Montmor's library, and struggling to tie together the two transfusion tubes, only five or six ounces of blood completed its journey from calf to man. But even this small amount seemed to have an effect, as Mauroy sweated and burned up in reaction. Judging that he'd had enough blood, Emmerez disentangled emittant and recipient, and closed up the wound in the man's arm. Servants helped Mauroy to bed to recover and returned to the library to clean up the carcass of the dead animal and mop up the spilled blood. They could hear the madman whistling and ranting in his room, though more faintly than before, until sleep overtook him.

When he awoke, he was calmer. Two days later, Denis and Emmerez put him through a second transfusion before a smaller audience, where the two men wouldn't be knocked about as they worked. This time Mauroy didn't put up quite so much of a fight as he was led into the library. Emmerez bled him of two ounces from his left arm and put another sixteen of calf's in. That was almost three times the amount of his first transfusion. His body reacted to the foreign blood again, and he sweated and ached and pleaded to be released. Denis ordered the connection between calf and man to be severed, and as Emmerez closed the wound Mauroy vomited up the contents of his stomach – bacon and fat – and continued to throw up what Denis described later as 'diverse liquors' for two hours before passing out from exhaustion.

Mauroy awoke once more and was now calm and alert. He called politely for a priest so he could confess his sins. The priest who came was, ironically enough, considering the species of Mauroy's donor, called Father Veau (French for 'veal'), and he could not believe what he had just seen. He came away from Mauroy's chamber amazed that he was no longer mad.

Denis wrote about this success in the same way he had with others, making sure its details were as widely known as possible. The *Journal des sçavans* published his letter, as usual, and an accurate translation of it even appeared in the Royal Society's *Transactions*. Sorbière, the secretary of Montmor's old academy and architect of its fall, heard about the transfusion success and got in touch with Denis. In the years since he had engineered the collapse of Académie Montmor, he'd

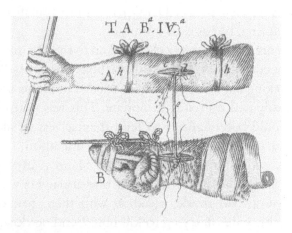

Figure 18 Italian blood transfusion, 1668.

fallen out with the prime minister and moved to Italy, where doctors were also trying their hand at transfusion. He wanted to know Denis's techniques, and everything about this new treatment for madness. The triumphant transfusionist replied with the descriptions asked of him, making sure Sorbière was in no doubt that they were performed at Montmor's home.

When Perrine came to reclaim her husband, she was over-joyed to find him sane again, though her approach was hesitant. According to Denis, Mauroy conducted himself 'with great presence of mind', relating his stories of naked rambling and arson, and finally told her about the transfu-sion. Denis wanted more time for observations, but Perrine took him home and did everything Denis advised her not to do. She fed him eggs and broth – two foods likely to heat his blood. And they had sex, also ill-advised because it, too, sup-posedly heated the blood. These were the reasons, or so it seemed, that Mauroy teetered back towards his old self again, and Perrine went to ask Denis for a third transfusion. He refused at first, but agreed eventually.

As Denis and Emmerez clattered up to the Mauroy house-hold in a coach, they noticed something was amiss. Mauroy was shrieking and wailing away as usual, but Denis spotted a calf already tied up ready to donate. This was unusual. The family could barely afford to feed themselves, let alone lay out all the equipment he'd need for the operation.

Denis and Emmerez approached Mauroy anyway, per-haps treading a little more gingerly than usual. He was in the middle of a mad tirade, pleading with them to stop, and accusing his wife of trying to kill him. Bending down at his side, working through his entreaties, they got out their lan-cets and prepared to make room for Mauroy's new dose of transplanted blood. But when they broke through his skin, he didn't bleed. Too many things out of the ordinary were happening, so Denis thought it best to pack up his instrument case and abandon the operation altogether. They left, the calf still tied up, untouched and still bleating away.

Mauroy died that night. Perrault, Lamy, Martinière and other transfusion detractors said it must have been the transfusion.

Martinière had, in the meantime, been publishing letters and papers about his extreme anti-transfusionist stance, sending them to prominent doctors, galvanizing them into action. His insistent outpourings were joined by many others, each taking a swipe at the interloping Montpellier transfusionist. The news travelled fast, reaching Louis XIV's secretary, who wrote to the Royal Society to say that Denis had discredited transfusion 'and no one will dare to try it in the future on men'. And only days after Mauroy's death, Lamy wrote a letter to his friend, proclaiming his own victory: 'the miserable adventure of the madman's death will be enough to overturn all of his beautiful imaginations and to ruin entirely his high hopes'.

Denis's reputation was in tatters once more. But the transfusion everybody thought had killed Mauroy hadn't even happened.

The calf and equipment, it seems, had been planted by hostile physicians. Perrine confessed as much when she turned up at Denis's door two months later, insisting some menacing doctors had surrounded her house and tried to bribe her into bearing false witness against Denis. She'd taken no money, she promised, but no sooner had Denis noted and thanked her for her confession than she suggested a tip would be a better way to say thanks. Denis shut the door on her.

The matter reached the courts. One document describes

how neighbours found 'certain Powders'. They'd also seen Perrine acting suspiciously, spoon in hand, feeding her husband, but going to a little too much trouble to telegraph to any onlookers that she was tasting the food before feeding it to him. In reality, she was tipping its contents onto the floor before bringing the spoon to her lips. The court concluded unanimously that Mauroy died of arsenic poisoning. Perrine was responsible, but the judge was convinced such a poor woman would not have acted alone. In a recently unearthed letter from a lawyer working on the case, Martinière and Lamy were named as part of a cabal against Denis.

The ruling was unanimous, and Denis was acquitted, but transfusion was effectively abandoned anyway. There's no indication the authorities actively banned it, but it was ruled that any future experiments would need the blessing of the Faculté de Médecine, and there was little chance of that ever happening. The Royal Society seems to have abandoned the operation, too, directing later research towards identifying the properties of blood. It would be a century and a half before anyone would transfuse blood again. Denis continued his research into blood, however, and in 1673 the Royal Society received yet another of his triumphant letters puffing a further success. They published this in *Philosophical Transactions* as 'Giving Notice of an Admirable Liquor, Instantly Stopping the Blood of Arteries Prickt or Cut . . .'. Denis had just invented styptic.

There would be no transplantation without an understanding of blood transfusion. The concept of spare-part surgery would be inconceivable without pumping hearts and circulating blood. And though the role and make-up of the blood itself remained a mystery to them, scientists like Lower and Denis still found mechanical ways to move it from one body to another. It would be only a short step from here to the idea that broken body parts could be replaced by 'spare', working parts. But seventeenth-century transfusions were never supposed to provide a replacement for lost blood. The blood itself, still entangled with ancient humoral and religious ideas, was rather a vehicle for something intangible and unquantifiable, like youth, meekness or strength. Despite this uncertainty about the blood, mechanical metaphors brought new ways of seeing ourselves as sets of connected components.

In the eighteenth century, the scientific spirit would flourish and everyday life would become more recognizably modern. The industrial and consumer revolutions brought another kind of transplant – the tooth transplant – which encapsulated the new superficiality of a time when body parts for transplant were given a cash value. Though they represented the latest in scientific medicine, the tooth transplants of the eighteenth century thrived because the poorest children in society were pressured into selling their newly erupted adult teeth to replace the rotting stumps of their social superiors. The eighteenth century was a low moral point for transplantation. It was also a time of crucial progress, as transplant operations emerged in an exciting new age of steam and money.

4. Teeth (1685–1803)

Jean-Baptiste Denis was still alive – in fact, he was only forty-two – when, in 1685, Charles Allen published instructions on how to transplant a tooth. Allen's book, *The Operator for the Teeth*, was also the first dentistry manual written in the English language, although the word 'dentist' didn't exist yet. The tooth transplant was very simple. A surgeon would strap down their recipient 'in some convenient place', tie their legs together and lodge open their mouth. Next to them, similarly restrained, would be a donor whose teeth best matched the size and shape of the recipient's. Allen offered a few suggestions for where a dentist might find suitable teeth: dogs, sheep, goats, or baboons. When ready, the surgeon would take his knife to the restrained baboon, say, carve out one of its teeth, leaving a bit of its gum still attached. He'd then, as quickly as possible, draw the patient's rotten tooth and immediately plug the gap with the baboon's. With time, the baboon's tooth and gum would knit itself into the patient's mouth. You *could* use another human as a donor, Allen advised, but this would be 'inhumane', since the 'reparation' of one mouth requires the 'ruine' of another. But 'I do not question in the least', Allen assured his readers, that whatever species the transplanted tooth came from, it 'would unite to the gums and jaw bone, and in a little time become as fast as the others'.[1]

We have no evidence that any baboons, dogs or goats ever graced Allen's dentist chair – or that he performed any transplants at all, for that matter – but when he was an apprentice, he witnessed something that persuaded him they would work. One day, he wrote, a lady came to see his master to have a tooth removed, convinced she had one too many. The old surgeon peered into her mouth and told her not to worry – she had the correct number of teeth. But she insisted there was an extra tooth. Inspecting her mouth again, he found it to be perfectly normal, but try as he might to convince her, she still pointed to the tooth – which she thought was growing on top of her other teeth – and demanded he take it out. So, no doubt causing a great deal of pain, Allen's master wrenched out the tooth she indicated only to pop it straight back in, presumably after first waving it in front of the woman's face for her edification. Within a few weeks, the replanted tooth had reunited with the woman's mouth.

Given the technical simplicity of the operation, it's probable that specialists like Allen transplanted teeth around this time, and maybe even earlier, though we have little hard evidence. The earliest confirmation we have of a tooth transplant is a foreign tooth lodged in a second-century skull, a single instance unearthed by archaeologists working in Ecuador. Otherwise we have only three references older than Allen's, and all are a little vague. The first is from eleventh-century Spain, where the Arabic physician Al-Zahrawi wrote, in passing, that teeth could be transplanted. The second is Henry VIII's regulations for barber surgeons, permitting them to implant teeth. The third is an allusion to a noble lady having a rotten tooth drawn and replaced with one from her maid's mouth.[2] The man who wrote about this final example in 1562, Ambroise Paré – a renowned French Renaissance surgeon famous for, amongst many other things, treating amputation wounds with a salve of egg yolk, rose oil and turpentine instead of the boiling oil more typical of the time – provided no detail.

Even if surgeons performed tooth transplants in extremis, the majority of the population relied on professional tooth *drawers*, whose remit was limited. As a licence granted in 1557 says, they were entitled to 'drawe teethe and to make cleane teethe and no more'.[3] A tooth drawer could be from any profession, from a clergyman to a jeweller to a wig maker.[4] In Figure 19, the tooth drawer is a farrier, depicted tugging at a woman's teeth with hoof nippers. She in turn tweaks his nose while her yokel family stand around pulling faces.

Charles Allen placed himself in another category altogether. He was no common tooth drawer, but an 'operator for the teeth'. He advised patients on hygiene, suggesting they brush their teeth once per week with a mixture of powdered coral, rose water and dragon's blood (a resin, for polish). And, in addition to the usual tooth pulling and cleaning, an operator for the teeth could fit false teeth made from walrus, elephant or hippopotamus ivory. Allen's tooth

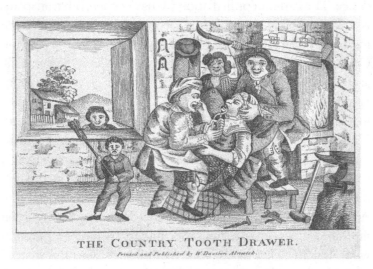

THE COUNTRY TOOTH DRAWER.
Printed and Published by W. Davison Alnwick.

Figure 19 'The Country Tooth-Drawer', after Richard Dighton.

transplant was, in fact, supposed to be a 'natural' alternative to the 'artificial' teeth he already provided.

Allen's vision of a future where animals sacrifice their teeth for the health of human mouths never came to pass. But in Paris, in the early years of the eighteenth century, the groundwork was laid for a boom in human–human tooth transplants.[5] It all started with Pierre Fauchard, then a navy surgeon. He wrote about one of his patients, a captain, who asked for a troublesome canine tooth to be removed. Not wanting to spoil his smile, though, he also asked if it could be replaced. Hoping the answer would be 'yes', he'd brought along one of the men under his command who would surrender his own canine. Luckily (for the officer, at least) Fauchard agreed. Inspecting the 'donor' tooth, however, he noticed it was too big for the captain's mouth, but he went ahead anyway, filing it down to be a better fit. The captain and his miserable companion marched out and Fauchard carried on with his day. 'Upon seeing him again eight years later', Fauchard wrote, 'the captain assured me that the transplanted tooth had lasted six years' before it decayed.

This modest success – and no doubt others like it – earned the tooth transplant a spot on a new menu of dental treatments devised by Fauchard in his two-volume *Le Chirurgien-dentiste, ou Traité des dents* ('The Dental Surgeon, or, Treatise on the Teeth'). Along with his tooth transplant, Fauchard also invented the ideas and tools for filling teeth, filing them and applying braces to straighten them. As well as these painfully familiar procedures, he included treatments that have thankfully since fallen out of favour, such as washing the mouth out with urine. This new kind of specialist surgeon he called a *dentiste*, and the name stuck, making its way into English as 'dentist' twenty years or so later.

Le Chirurgien-dentiste was, to dentistry, what Vesalius's *Fabrica* was to anatomy, and within its field was just as important. The book outlined a new scientific approach to treating teeth that relied on experimentation and observation. And just as Vesalius had no interest in slavishly repeating flawed ancient Greek anatomy, Fauchard set out to rid tooth care of its own superstitions, its own literal demons. One of the most common causes of tooth decay at the time was supposedly a tiny creature called a tooth worm that would find its way inside your teeth. It would wriggle around, nibbling on your pulp until it caused ecstatic, sharp, throbbing pain so unbearable it would send you in agonized tears to the tooth drawer to have the offending worm pulled out, tooth and all.

The tooth worm is one of those phenomena – like the association between blood and life and the idea that skin behaves like tree bark – seemingly shared across cultural and geographical boundaries and throughout the entirety of human history. The Cherokee reported toothache as 'a mere worm that has wrapped itself round the base of the tooth'. The native word for 'toothache' in Madagascar – many miles from Cherokee territory – means 'poorly through the worm', and an ancient Egyptian papyrus from 1200–1100 BC tells a story about a bureaucrat stuck at a desert outpost complaining 'the worm gnaweth at his teeth'.[6] Leo Kanner, a German doctor and dental historian (he was also the man to name 'autism' as a medical condition) printed a sketch of Bitoso the Fasting, the 'toothache demon' of the Bosnian Gypsies. Bitoso is a worm with three heads, one of nine demon-children of Ana the fairy queen and the dwarf King Loçolica. Kanner rather adorably described him as the 'least harmful' demon of all.[7]

The tooth worm even has an origin story. The dental historian Malvin E. Ring, in his illustrated history of dentistry, shows a clay tablet from Babylonia that tells the story of the tooth worm's creation:

After Anu [had created heaven] . . .
The earth had created the rivers,
The rivers had created the canals,
The canals had created the marsh,
The marsh had created the worm.
The worm went weeping, before Shamash,
His tears flowing before Ea:
'What wilt thou give me for my sucking?'
'I shall give thee the ripe fig and the apricot.'
'Of what use are they to me, the ripe fig and the apricot?
'Lift me up and among the teeth
'And the gums cause me to dwell!
'The blood of the tooth will I suck,
'And of the gum will I gnaw the roots!'[8]

Out of one historical mouth and into another, the tooth worm seemed to wriggle its way around the globe. Remedies for tooth worms ranged from spitting salt on fresh graves to kissing donkeys, but the only way to drive them out for sure would be to employ a tooth drawer. Then, in 1728, with his scientific approach to operating on teeth, Fauchard vanquished the worm, challenging its existence simply on the grounds that he'd never seen one and couldn't find one, even with a microscope, no matter how hard he looked. If by any chance tooth worms did exist, he concluded, he doubted they had anything to do with tooth decay or toothache. That was most probably down to mundane matters like malnutrition and sugar consumption, by both of which early eighteenth-century France was particularly afflicted. A series of wars, epidemics and failed harvests had brought death to many and malnutrition, and therefore bad teeth, to most others. Even the head of the Académie Royale des Sciences, Louis XIV himself – who was, by 1700, in his sixties – had already been completely toothless for twenty years.[9] His dental problems resulted more from his sweet tooth than undernourishment, but even with the best treatment money could buy, tooth care was effectively limited to rubbing them down with a cloth. And here was Fauchard, insisting that dental woes were caused not by invisible and unstoppable little worms, but were instead identifiable and fixable problems. With the promise of dental care more suited to image-conscious nobles, Paris – and then the rest of Europe – soon had two distinct kinds of tooth-care specialist.

The first had an extremely long history – the tooth drawer, who, until Fauchard, was the only option. In eighteenth-century Paris, tooth drawers were often actors, performers, charlatans from Italy who would excise troublesome teeth as a kind of street theatre. One such artist flicked out troublesome teeth from the back of his horse using the point of a sword blade. Another clamped his thumb and forefinger onto even the most stubborn teeth and pulled them out to the accompaniment of violins and dancing girls. The Pont Neuf in Paris was a popular spot for such capers, and the resultant hullabaloo would have been the backdrop for Jean-Baptiste's public transfusion from dog to dog alongside the same bridge in 1667. Well into the eighteenth century, too, travelling medicine men plied their trade on that famous crossing, with the most sought-after spot just in front of the equestrian statue of Henri IV at its very centre.

For much of the first half of the eighteenth century, a man called Jean Thomas, or 'Le Grand Thomas', as he was more commonly known on account of his sheer size, took pride of place next to this statue. His portrait shows a man beplumed. Peacock feathers cascaded from his oversized tri-corn hat, and a sabre with a handle shaped like an eagle poked out of his pocket. He would stand, every day, shel-tered under the roof a wheeled platform, at one corner of which dangled a giant tooth ('Gargantua's awesome molar'). At another corner there was a bell he'd ring when touting for business. When it pealed, and his voice boomed over the marketplace chatter, crowds would gather around him. And then, as the dramatist Louis-Sébastien Mercer put it when reminiscing about seeing Thomas during his childhood, 'toothache seemed to expire at his feet'.

For all his rustic showmanship, Le Grand Thomas had a licence from the Paris College of Surgery, and had served the army with his tooth pulling. His treatments were even certi-fied by the king's premier physician, though what he – or any other tooth puller – could offer was scarcely different from that suffered by the rest of the population.[10] Physicians would still not dirty their hands with surgery, and delving into a stinking mouth was a particularly low form of that art, which, the royal surgeon Pierre Dionis commented in 1708, 'smacks of the charlatan and the mountebank'. Ungenerous sentiments like this passed so far into the public conscious-ness that, as the historian Colin Jones wrote, 'to lie like a tooth puller' was a common phrase in the French language.

Fauchard used this reputation, along with his scientific credentials and book (which he was canny enough to dedi-cate to the king's premier surgeon) to set himself up as the second kind of tooth-care specialist: a dentist – a genteel, understated alternative to the dancing girls and jugglers. Some tooth pullers are fine human beings, he conceded, offering a much-needed service with specialist knowledge of the mouth. Others, though, live up to the stereotype of being liars and tricksters. 'Some say that they cure toothache by particular essences,' he wrote, 'others by plasters; others by prayers and the sign of the cross.' Others, he added, 'have specifics to kill the worms that they imagine are gnawing the tooth'. He, on the other hand, set himself up in a discreet surgery on the Left Bank, not far from the Pont Neuf, where a more discerning patient could visit in private.

Scientific credentials and the promise of restrained, effective treatment attracted a new kind of client wanting to achieve a smile appropriate to their social position. Some of these would have been aristocratic, but Fauchard would also have appealed to those who wanted to *become* a 'person of quality', the kinds of people who fuelled a recent boom in books about civility and manners. He appealed directly to this discerning public's sense of decorum and etiquette by referring to the 'appearance of the mouth', and even the 'appearance of the voice' as something ladies and gentlemen find 'of principal concern' when 'speaking or making music in public'. With a growth in venues like coffee houses, parks and promenades there were also more opportunities to see and be seen, to smile and be smiled at. And these people who might have desired a presentable mouth were certainly not the same people who would prefer to visit the country tooth drawer. Fauchard would have offered the tooth transplant as one of the many ways these wealthy few could keep smiling as the years advanced.

Still, transplanting teeth would remain a tiny part of a dentist's repertoire, performed in exceptional circumstances. At least for now. But when Fauchard wrote his book, the Western world was on the cusp of transforming in two important ways. The first was a revolution in science and medicine, which would convince people that their body parts were interchangeable, that they were all made of the same stuff. The second promised the opposite: new ideas about personal identity convinced people they were individuals, and they sought to curate and assert their individuality. These two great shifts were wrapped up in the industrial revolution and the consumer revolution that accompanied it. Respected scientists would champion the tooth transplant as a viable operation. And society would create a demand for healthy, white teeth, and a supply of those desperate enough to part with them.

We're All the Same

Between 1730 and 1735, as Pierre Fauchard mingled with well-to-do Parisians, an ailing Dutch physician and medical educator called Herman Boerhaave was performing his final lecture series in Leiden, planting an intellectual seed that would eventually lead to the first tooth transplants backed by science.[11] Where most physicians would still have cited bad blood and imbalanced humours as the most likely cause of disease, in these lectures – 206 in total – Boerhaave blamed the nervous system. Like his predecessors, he thought the nerves were hollow, and that what he called 'subtle juices' filled with sub-microscopic 'animal spirits' flowed through them. When these flowed freely, you were healthy, but when they became blocked or frustrated you would get a nervous disease. Disturbances in the nervous system were everywhere in Boerhaave's medical system. Almost any ailment, in fact, could be considered 'nervous'. Not only did nervous disorder cover all mental conditions, but also anything that came under the categories of vertigo, apoplexy or epilepsy. Even blindness and deafness he counted amongst nervous diseases, as well as toothache, some infections and a few skin complaints involving inflamed nerve endings. The nerves were so important to Boerhaave's understanding of human anatomy that in his seventy-seventh lecture, he referred to the body as *machina nervosa* – the nervous machine.

For William Harvey and his followers, transfusion had been a matter of moving blood through tubes and transplanting whatever magical spirit was inside. Boerhaave's nervous machine drew on many of the same influences. He'd studied Vesalius, knew chemistry and combined this knowledge with the work of individual trailblazers like Harvey and Boyle. Then he'd combine all of this with the teachings of ancient Greek physicians to come up with his own ideas about the mechanical and chemical composition of the body. He seemed to pick from every branch of the tree of knowledge – every branch, that is, but medicine, from which he plucked only a single fruit: Hippocrates. When Boerhaave had been a student, he'd attended hardly any lectures, and instead read ancient medical writers in chronological order. But since Hippocrates was the earliest source – and therefore, to Boerhaave, the purest – he had little time for other bodies of medical work. Boerhaave only ever referred to one other medical writer in the whole of his career, the English physician Thomas Sydenham (or, as he's also known, 'the English Hippocrates'[12]). But by engaging deeply with anatomy and science, Boerhaave conceived of a body that was an almost entirely material, chemical object – made of solids that contained liquids and gases, one that could be understood and treated in terms of weights, forces and hydrostatic pressure. The *machina nervosa* was the most comprehensively mechanical body yet.

This material, measurable body was, however, complicated by Boerhaave's Christian faith. His first degree was in theology, in fact, and he didn't intend to become a physician at all. Even after his medical degree he wanted to become a minister, but his chances were scuppered by what historians refer to as an 'incident' on a *trekschuit* – a horse-pulled canal boat used for public transport. The story goes that he over-heard some animated passengers denouncing the philosopher Baruch Spinoza. Spinoza had been excommunicated and ostracized twenty-odd years earlier for claiming that God was not an individual deity but the totality of existence. Boerhaave doubted his loud-mouthed fellow passengers were doing anything but braying mindless objections, so he challenged them to explain themselves. When they couldn't, and the sounds of their brash indignation were replaced by the lapping of water on the side of the boat, a nameless pas-senger took down Boerhaave's name. His dream of being a churchman was left in tatters. But he never lost faith, and he found a place for it in his medical system. His belief in God and unshakeable conviction in an immaterial soul, when applied to mechanical philosophy, gave him *esprits de cerveau* – an immaterial, God-given soul, which occupied the body – and the *sensorium commune*, a point of connection between the body and that Christian spirit.

The *sensorium commune* is the part of the brain where, as its name suggests, all the nerves converge, the point where grey matter meets white matter. For Boerhaave it was where 'you', as a Christian soul, sat and dispatched instructions for the rest of your body to follow. If you willed your legs to cross, for instance, the *sensorium commune* would send instructions through the tentacle-like nerves threading throughout your body and they would comply, as if there was a little person sat in your head pulling levers.

Boerhaave is remembered today as the first medical man

to take teaching to the patient's bedside. His influence in medical education is vast, and for this his memory is still held dear in Leiden.[13] For the story of transplant surgery it was the 'nervous machine' that would have the most influence. When he died in 1737, his adoring students would develop increasingly extreme theories that would result in the first scientific justification for performing tooth transplants.

The first radical position taken by Boerhaave's students was derived from his notion that the body was composed of solids, liquids and gases and that its workings could be understood in mechanical and chemical terms. Some of Boerhaave's students and admirers were doing away with the Christian dimension of his system even as he lay on his death bed in Leiden. Quite soon, some were able to argue that we may not have souls at all and could be completely self-contained. From such an extreme mechanism, it would in the future be possible to disassociate people from their parts – if body parts don't necessarily belong to a particular person, they could in theory be given to another.

The second line of research – vitalism – also extended directly from Boerhaave's nervous machine and attempted to account for the soul and life itself. Vitalism is a conviction that life is a thing or principle, as opposed to the result of physical or chemical processes, and so lends itself very well to talk of souls and spirits. As a general belief, it's ancient and widespread. Galen's belief that the 'divine breath' of life finds its way into the body through the lungs is a vitalist conviction, as are animistic beliefs of souls and spirits inhabiting bodies. But vitalism doesn't have to be religious or spiritual. And despite Boerhaave's Christian beliefs, his students often described their vitalist ideas in material terms, with life being an unfathomably intricate, even invisible function of the body. Dentists would come to rely on certain eighteenth-century vitalist convictions, making them integral to tooth transplantation, providing a convincing (though erroneous) explanation for why one body part adheres to another: a 'vital principle', 'spirit' or 'spark' brings life to it.

Man, a Machine

René Descartes had already written that animals were nothing but machines, but it was possible that the same could be said of humans. This was the position of the philosopher and physician Julien Offray de La Mettrie – one of Boerhaave's doting students, who also translated many of his teacher's works into French. Like Boerhaave, La Mettrie started life wanting to go into the ministry, but in the end he made the decidedly impious move to turn the *machina nervosa* into the full-on *l'homme machine* – the machine man.

Industrialists and inventors of the time made it easy for La Mettrie to cultivate an extreme mechanist bent. They showed it was possible to imitate and even improve the function of the human body by artificial means. The French inventor Jacques de Vaucanson was a particularly important influence on him. In February 1738, Vaucanson shared a stage in Paris with a flautist he'd built.[14] A paying crowd had gathered in the since-demolished Hôtel de Longueville to hear the music and watch as Vaucanson gave a guided tour of the flautist's innards. Taking ten to fifteen people at a time, the inventor led his audience to his wooden colleague, which he'd carved and painted white to mimic the Lyonese sculptor Antoine Coysevox's marble statue of a faun playing a flute. He opened up the automaton's chest cavity, showing off nine bellows. By activating these in different combinations, Vaucanson had created a kind of mechanical lung, which he could programme to simulate breath. Then, with moving metal lips and tongue, he could manipulate the air flow onto the flute's mouthpiece, interrupting and modifying it now and then to change pitch as a human musician would. The robot was technically impressive and elegant, but its value wasn't derived solely from its inventor's solutions to such mechanical difficulties. Most people of the time still associated breath directly with life. They thought it contained one of the three Aristotelian or Galenic souls, the animal spirit drawn from divine breath, through the lungs. Within a few puffs, and a couple of toots, this ancient source of life, spirit, soul, had been brought down to earth and exposed as a mere bodily function.

With the breath of life now imitated, Vaucanson made the slender wooden fingers rise and fall over the finger holes in sequence. The joints were fixed to substitute tendons, with four chains lifting the four fingers. The flautist could in this way play twelve tunes for the audience's pleasure. It took Vaucanson a while to figure out how to get the sound just right. Perhaps it was the mechanist's imagination, but although the notes and the intervals between them were accurate, the sound was cold and spiritless. Listening to the tap of wood, he puzzled over his most virtuosic and uncanny performer. Then, playing Geppetto to the flautist's Pinocchio, Vaucanson tacked some skin – that is, leather – over the automaton's fingertips. With an organic interface now covering the finger holes, the tapping stopped and the music came to life.

Vaucanson's flute player showed that even something so deeply human as making music could be reduced to a matter of mechanics. A year later, in 1739, he would push further. This time, his flute player was accompanied by two more robots. The first would become Vaucanson's most famous machine: a fully mechanical and articulated duck. On a pedestal next to the life-size flute player, it was tiny – the size of a real duck, in fact – but plated in gold-coloured copper. It was so heavily engineered it moved just like the real thing, drinking, quacking, splashing water around with its beak. Its mechanist creator had installed over 400 articulated parts in each wing, so it could also preen itself like a real duck. It would even gobble grain out of Vaucanson's hand, gulping it down with a realistic swish of its robotic neck. And, to the delight of his audience, the duck even seemed to digest the grain and poo it out in front of them. The digestion was actually an illusion. The duck did eat, but the digestion process was too complex to mimic in tubes and valves, so Vaucanson created ready-made poo in a specially constructed compartment. Crowds delighted in the creature. Voltaire wrote that without Vaucanson's shitting duck we'd have nothing to remind us of the glory of France.

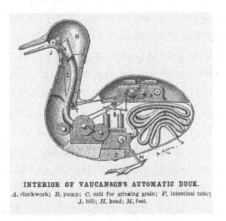

INTERIOR OF VAUCANSON'S AUTOMATIC DUCK.
A, clockwork; *B*, pump; *C*, mill for grinding grain; *F*, intestinal tube; *J*, bill; *H*, head; *M*, feet.

Figure 20 Imaginary rendering of Vaucanson's digesting duck in *Scientific American*, 1899.

The pooing duck stole the show, robbing the audience's attention from Vaucanson's second new automaton, a musician dressed like a dancing shepherd who piped out a repertoire of twenty minuets, rigadoons and country dances on a pipe and drum. The relative simplicity of these instruments may have made this new automaton a little less impressive, at least on first sight, but the mechanics were even more complicated than those of his flautist. The musician would have struck the drum at different intensities and speeds, which required unfathomably intricate mechanics. The piper didn't need such complicated breath control as the flautist, but it piped out melodies impossible for human fingers. Not only could mechanics reproduce human and animal actions, Vaucanson showed, they could improve on them.[15]

A couple of years after displaying his trinity of flautist, piper and duck, Vaucanson found himself at the receiving end of the working man's ire for suggesting that machines could improve their craftwork.[16] He'd been favoured by Louis XV, who charged him with improving France's silk manufacture, which was starting to trail behind that of England. A proud nation like France could not allow this, and if Vaucanson could create mechanical musicians to better human ones, perhaps he could do the same for textile manufacturers. He accepted the challenge and came up with the Vaucanson loom, a forerunner of the Jacquard loom, which wove the finest patterns and most complex designs. The operator was now a mere slave to the machine, needing only to feed it with hole-punched paper and pull a few levers. French textile workers, realizing that such an invention would put them out of work, responded to their feared obsolescence by throwing stones at Vaucanson when they saw him in the street.

A similar backlash occurred in Britain after the introduction of the flying shuttle – the metal-tipped bullet that gave the textile factory its characteristic and unrelenting soundscape, clack-clack, dum-m, clack-clack, dum-m. A mob descended on the home of its inventor, John Kay. If a mural

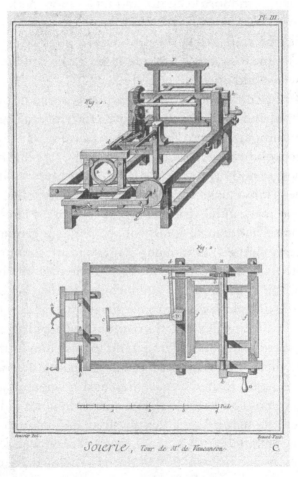

Figure 21 Vaucanson's loom, from Diderot and D'Alembert's *Encyclopédie*, 1762–73.

by Ford Madox Brown in Manchester town hall is to be believed, Kay was smuggled out of his own house wrapped in a carpet. But there would be no midnight retreats for Vaucanson. The automaton maker was unapologetic to say the least, and responded by insisting that 'a horse, an ox or an ass can make cloth more beautiful and much more perfect than the most able silk workers'. And, as an extra two-fingered salute to the craftspeople, he proved it by programming one of his looms to weave a baroque floral fabric and built it to be powered and operated by a donkey.

Drawing confidence from Vaucanson – whom he called 'a new Prometheus' – La Mettrie wrote a tract called 'L'homme machine' in 1747, arguing that, if this mechanist could breathe life into wood and metal, it might also be the case that human beings were nothing but machines. *L'homme machine* not only had mechanical lungs and heart, though – everything about him was mechanical, from sinew to synapse. Harvey, the infusionists and transfusionists of the previous century, and Boerhaave himself all thought some kind of soul or spirit inhabited a carnal contraption. La Mettrie took the human mechanism to the extreme, and included intelligence, sensation, consciousness, memory and imagination as part of the machinery.[17] Any human action or function could, in theory, be recreated with nuts and bolts, and to push him further La Mettrie challenged Vaucanson to make a 'talker'. It would be more complex than the machines he'd made to date but should be possible in theory. (The mechanist never did make a 'talker', though by 1771 the physician and poet Erasmus Darwin, grandfather of Charles, was tinkering with leather, silk ribbons and bellows and produced a rudimentary, croaking mechanical voice box. He made it say 'mamma, papa, map, and pam'. With more time, he wrote, he thought a giant version of his machine might one day 'command an army or instruct a crowd'[18]).

Some accused La Mettrie of downgrading humans to the level of Vaucanson's automata, a brute machine with no intelligence or soul.[19] But this, he was clear, was not what he meant at all. He was a doctor who just wanted to see the *truth* of the body so he could treat it properly. Science and scientific medicine were, he felt, supposed to show the world as it was, and to make our own reality an exception to this rule would be vanity. Though some found it difficult to swallow, La Mettrie's view seems to have won out, and throughout the eighteenth century, anatomists busied themselves by sticking their hands into corpses, scribbling down what they saw, felt and even tasted. These explorers of the body would map it to the millimetre, uncovering and charting bodily functions, seeking ever more precise descriptions of the human machine, and in an analogue to empire, raced to claim parts and name them after themselves. By the end of the century it wasn't unusual to find a common physician who invested themselves in the materialist line. Samuel Taylor Coleridge was even able to complain in 1796 of doctors, who are 'shallow animals, having always employed their minds about Body and Gut, they imagine that in the whole system of things there is nothing but Gut and Body'.[20] By the time Coleridge wrote this, the idea that people were nothing but complex collections of mechanical parts had become commonplace and (more or less) uncontroversial.

Meanwhile, other naturalists and scientists were starting to discover that living creatures could *not* be machines after all – at least not the nuts-and-bolts kind. In the late 1730s the Belgian naturalist Abraham Trembley was the tutor to the sons of Comte de Bentinck near The Hague in the Netherlands.[21] After

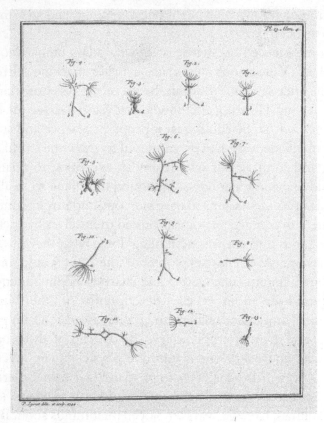

Figure 22 Engraving of Trembley's polyps, 1744.

a few years settling into his employment, he started to explore the nobleman's grounds. He acquired a microscope – a device invented over a century earlier, but which had recently been dramatically improved – and used it to look at samples from the ponds in his employer's estate. The seemingly stagnant water was teeming. Larger specimens drew his interest, such as the freshwater coelenterate hydra – the freshwater polyp.

The tiny animal was shaped like a reed and looked to be

made of a gelatinous substance. At one end it had a hollow, mouth-like opening, and it seemed to reproduce through a series of shoots. It looked like a plant and had in fact been classified as such by the pioneering microscopist Antonie van Leeuwenhoek in 1703. But Trembley noticed that it acted more like an animal than any plant he'd seen, with its ability to propel itself by contracting and extending, and a strange arm-like structure near its mouth that reached out for prey. Trembley chopped bits off these polyps and watched them fuse together again. If he put them close enough to one another, he could even get parts from two unrelated polyps to join together into a completely new animal. And if he chopped a polyp into two and kept them apart, they would duplicate themselves and he'd be left with two animals where he'd previously had only one.

When he made his discovery public, it so went against mainstream opinion that no one believed him. The world, he complained, was full of *les incrédules*. So he made a do-it-yourself kit complete with polyps and instructions on how you could make your own chimera. One of his kits went to the Royal Society in London, which demonstrated it to an audience of 120 and published his findings in their *Transactions* in 1743. A few years later the Italian priest and biologist Lazzaro Spallanzani pointed out that other small animals seemed to have powers of regeneration – snails, frog larvae and salamanders. And, inspired by Trembley's findings, the Genevan naturalist Charles Bonnet mounted his own experiments and showed how worms had similar regenerative powers to polyps.[22] 'How lucky is the earthworm', one German commentator wrote, 'to whom are allotted ... an infinite number of souls ... meanwhile we poor star-gazers must sourly drag along with only one solitary soul.' If an entire animal could sprout from a single part, or some animals could simply grow new parts, then surely, they could not be machines. Descartes never would have dreamed, Bonnet's commentator went on to say, that the animals he thought to be automata actually have so many souls they 'crowd out the human race'.[23]

Trembley's observations didn't seem to fit the mechanistic view being promoted by people like La Mettrie. But La Mettrie had an answer to the question of regenerating animals that actually strengthened his own conviction in a mechanical, material body: he asked, 'Does it not contain within itself the causes which produce its regeneration?'[24] There is no need for God or a soul, in other words, because the polyp shows that matter can clearly organize and multiply by itself. The implication of discovering these regenerating animals was that, if this literal pond life can regenerate, it should be possible also for so-called 'higher' animals like humans to do the same. It turned out humans *are* capable of the kind of regeneration we see in polyps, salamanders and worms, although it would take until the late twentieth century for scientists to find such a mechanism in stem cells. But even by the mid-eighteenth century, at least for La Mettrie, it was conceivable that humans lacked souls. Perhaps, in other words, the body is all we have, and all that distinguishes us from one another is an illusion.

A Vital Spark

Alongside the evolving mechanist position, vitalists began to become more and more convinced that there was a mysterious life force inside the body – a force that would soon become an essential component in convincing dental surgeons that tooth transplants worked. Most of the vitalist research stemmed from Edinburgh – a university where

Boerhaave was so influential that when the medical school there was founded in 1726, the professors of both theory and practice of medicine as well as the professors of medicine and chemistry had all been his pupils. Robert Whytt, for example, the professor of medicinal theory, stuck fairly closely to his teacher's ideas when he proposed that the nervous system, along with an 'active sentient principle' (or soul), was responsible for sensation and movement. Having such a 'principle' shackled life to the body, and even specifically located it in the nerves.[25] Whytt's arch-rival, the Swiss naturalist Albrecht von Haller – yet another of Boerhaave's pupils – felt broadly the same, but thought that muscles didn't need the nerves, soul or sensation to contract and jerk about. They were 'irritable' because they responded to being prodded and pricked, but they weren't 'sensible' like the nerves.[26]

Within fifty years of this kind of materialistic vitalism, it was possible to believe that life itself might be a physical, material thing that constantly moved around the body and stopped when you died. Some doctors and scientists even thought that, if you were quick enough, you could bring someone back to life by encouraging their apparently dormant vital principle to get back on the move. The physician William Cullen put such an idea into practice when he devised a way to revive drowned people.[27] Although the heart, lung and circulation of the blood support life, Cullen wrote in a public-minded letter to Lord Cathcart in 1776, it doesn't necessarily mean life has gone when they stop. A 'vital principle' is active in bodies, and though it might be weak, could be revived again along with the heart and lungs. He goes through some standard methods for trying to revive the drowned – hanging them upside down by the heels, standing them on their head, rolling them over a barrel – and rejects them all.

Even if the drowned did revive after being mistreated like this, the pressure such treatment caused might burst blood vessels in the brain or lungs.

The longer the body has been in the water, the colder it will be and the weaker its life force. But, Cullen suggests, if it hasn't been in there for too long and is still warm with vital heat, the best course of action is to 'agitate' it. You might need to carry it to a warm place, holding it flat with the head slightly raised. Next, strip the body of its wet clothes and wrap it in warm blankets. Once it's dry, he suggests clothing it with the shirt or waistcoat taken from a living person. He goes on to suggest more ways of warming a body, from giving it a warm bath, to rubbing it, to covering it with warm sand, to climbing in bed with it and pressing your naked body against it. And since the intestines are the most 'irritable', he recommends 'forcing a quantity of air into them by the fundament'. Or even better, apply 'the smoke of burning tobacco'. He recommended a device to administer this air or smoke, which he

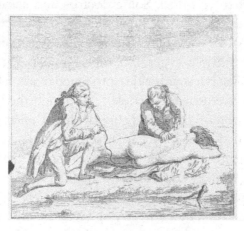

Figure 23 Two men attempting to resuscitate a drowned woman by blowing into her anus, 1774.

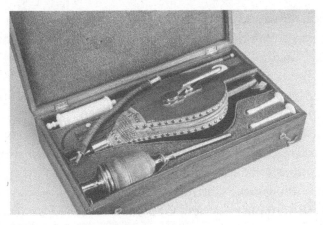

Figure 24 Resuscitation set, Europe, 1801–50.

thought should be in every doctor's bag and readily available near all bodies of water. Quite a few of these still exist in science and medicine museums around the world. They consist of a pair of bellows to pump air or smoke up somebody's bottom to 'animate' their 'vital principle'. If you can't find a pair of these bellows, Cullen suggests that at a pinch you could blow the smoke through a common tobacco pipe, aimed directly at the intestines.

Although mechanism and vitalism are traditionally presented as opposites, some mechanists and vitalists seemed to agree in one crucial way: the body is a material, earth-bound thing. It is easy to see how this is the case for a mechanist, who sees bodies as combinations of components, with no need for any kind of soul. But vitalists have often *embraced* the idea of a soul. The new 'nervous' vitalism bound the soul to the body, though, and made it into a material thing that pulsed through it. This could be a Christian soul, as it was for Boerhaave, but it didn't need to be. It could be a mere particle. As medical belief in souls and humours declined even further, more and more doctors became convinced that the body was a material thing. This meant more effective, standardized medical treatment, which was generally very good news. But it was also increasingly looking like we were losing our sense of individuality, or at least our sense that our bodies were unquestionably ours alone.

The trend towards a material conception of the body was accompanied by a social and cultural revolution that seemed to counteract the loss of our inherent individuality. In this century, along came Christmas pantomime, coffee-house culture and shopping – a new, Georgian society of excitement and inequality, of industry, money and social difference. This new world gave us fresh ways to be unique, a way to *construct* and *buy* our own identities and to assert ourselves through our possessions. When this was combined with the pressure of scientists and doctors increasingly seeing bodies as material things, for a short time at least, it became possible to buy other people's body parts and claim them as our own.

It's All About Me

From quite early in the eighteenth century, 'nervousness' became something of a medical trope, and 'nervous diseases' a peculiar obsession with the English middle classes. Some doctors tried to use the classification of nervous diseases to convince their patients they were special. George Cheyne, not a particularly well-known or brilliant doctor, wrote *The English Malady* in 1733, which became a moderately famous book about the nerves and nervousness.[28] Nervous disorders only attacked people from the upper classes, he wrote, 'the brightest and most spiritual, and whose Genius is most keen and penetrating'.[29] His conviction in the natural superiority of the upper classes was so strong he thought one third of all upper-class disorders were 'nervous'. Presumably, by associating their diseases with their social status Cheyne guaranteed himself a nice flow of wealthy patients happy to be comforted that their illnesses were superior, and their superiority was, moreover, a natural, biological fact (and that their gout had nothing whatsoever to do with their overindulgence).

Nerves and nervous disorders persisted amongst the upper classes throughout the century. You just need to look through a few Jane Austen novels to find the ineffectual, fan-fluttering victims of nervousness. And it could be serious. In Samuel Richardson's 1748 best-seller *Clarissa*, readers work their way through nearly a million words of story to find out that Clarissa dies because of her 'weak Nerves'.

The working classes, on the other hand, had no such diseases. As the upper classes were indulged in their senses of superiority and nervousness, most people were, in fact, becoming more mechanized and downtrodden. The textile industry alone, in the decade 1764–74, welcomed three revolutionary developments – the Spinning Jenny, the Water Frame and the Spinning Mule. In 1774 James Watt moved to Birmingham to work with the manufacturer Matthew Boulton. Soon, the two men would sell their first steam engine – the technological successor to the Newcomen engine. In these decades and beyond, manufacture would mechanize further and further, and manufacturers and industrialists would aim to increase production and personal profits at the cost of the reduced wages and living standards of their workers. In industry, the working man became more like a machine, just as in Vaucanson's hands machine became more like man.

Such men and women were too indelicate and lumpen to

have nervous disorders. An interesting spin on this came much later, in 1807, when the doctor Thomas Trotter – described in the frontispiece to his book as the 'late physician to His Majesty's fleet' – wrote that nervous complaints were now common amongst the lower classes, too. Puffing out his patriotic chest, he concluded that this must have been because of Britain's 'peculiar situation'; its climate, its free government, political institutions and vast wealth meant that a better standard of living was 'so diffused among all ranks of people'.[30] Now everyone had the good fortune to be nervous.

Another manifestation of our growing individuality was the way we started to identify ourselves with our worldly goods. In the thirteenth century, for instance, St Thomas Aquinas was disturbed by the theological ramifications of having hair and nails. Were they really part of his body? It certainly seemed that way, but he shed and cut them, so maybe it would be more accurate to say they were something his body excreted, not really bits of him at all? His teeth fell into the same category, he thought – a part of his body, but somehow not *really*.[31] If God considered his eyebrows, fingernails and teeth to be tantamount to waste products, would poor Thomas Aquinas be resurrected bald, with an empty mouth, unable to scratch himself? Such a question would have been irrelevant, even laughable, for most people by the eighteenth century.

The fact that hair, nails and teeth were once considered superfluous to a person's identity tells us something about how different our senses of self are now. To describe this social change on a grander scale, in the eighteenth century we went from seeing ourselves as *essences* to seeing ourselves as *compositions*. Just a century earlier, people were afraid that blood transfusions and skin grafts might alter who they inescapably were, change their predestined and pre-designed selves. By the eighteenth century, the philosopher David Hume could convincingly argue that there is no such thing as the permanent self anyway, and that our identities are not fixed. Historians have referred to this shift as 'individuation' because we evolved a more-or-less modern understanding of what it means to be an individual.[32] And 'individuation' was linked to industry, to money, to property.

No longer so deeply concerned with our souls and instead understanding our bodies in ever more mechanical terms, it seemed we weren't so different from one another after all. Even those of us degraded by increasingly mindless factory work evolved a new sense of uniqueness, new ways of finding and expressing individuality. We bought more and associated our selves with our belongings. We began to build our identities around our possessions or lack of them.[33] With a cherrywood Chippendale side chair here, a silver tea set there, we showed off our tastes to anyone who would pay attention. In this way we started to construct our own identities, replacing the divine essences we lost.

It would take many years for the masses to acclimatize themselves to the idea, but people began to judge one another by what they owned. Over the coming decades – even centuries – we declared louder and louder that we are all individuals. Josiah Wedgwood said that he populated his factories with 'such machines of Men as cannot err',[34] a sentiment that seems to encapsulate the man-machine at its least human and least humane. But Wedgwood was in the business of making and selling pots – beautiful, meaningful, life-enhancing objects that people shopped for, treasured and bragged about. Instead of finding yourself within yourself, you found yourself in pots like his, as well as pipes, buttons, sideboards, chairs, the family silver.

If the question Thomas Aquinas asked – 'What parts of my body are me?' – is an old-fashioned one, a more consumerist society might ask, 'What parts of my body do I own?' Or, 'Who owns my body?' In the eighteenth century, it even became common to buy and sell body parts. Arms, legs, heads, even entire bodies – either unfettered or prepared by expert hands – began to be worth money as medical men and students bought anatomical specimens as learning aids.[35] The physician William Hunter, along with his brother, John, produced and collected vast numbers of preparations like these. One of my favourite cartoons, from 1782, shows his anatomy museum on Windmill Street in London on the day of the resurrection. To one side of him, a pair of skeletons are reacquainting – 'My dear madam', one says, 'I hope you are well. I am overjoyed to see you' – and to the other, two corpses are fighting over a leg. Hunter is in the middle, having never supposed such a day would come, with an old woman at one side, asking him to return her 'virgin honour' that he 'corked up' in one of his specimen jars. By the eighteenth century, some could even see the resurrection as a matter of property, of who owns what. It shows how, in some circles, 'Who am I?' and 'What do I own?' became so close as to be almost indistinguishable.

The emergence of fashion in the

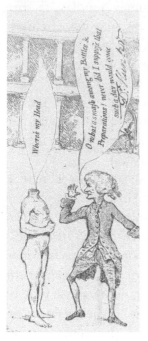

Figure 25 'The Resurrection: or an Internal view of the Museum in Windmill Street on the Last Day' (detail).

eighteenth century was also related to this novel tendency to associate oneself with one's belongings. Although there were – and still are – exceptions, we stopped working ourselves up into a tizz about the theological status of our toenails, hair and teeth, but worried how these things looked, smelt and felt. Whole shop-salon empires sprang up, dedicated to the pimping of said hair, nails and teeth. Then, as now, we were 'worth it', able to escape ourselves by adopting a new look. It'd been almost a complete reversal of the situation Aquinas worried about: it doesn't much matter what's on the inside, as long as the outside is well curated.

We also dressed to make a statement, from patterned silks to stiff corsets. By the middle of the century, spectacles were no longer just a sign of poor vision, they started to connote intelligence. False legs and wigs became more popular, too – ways of shaping a body its owner needn't be ashamed of.[36] Together with industry and rampant capitalism, such new ways of designing your individuality according to your financial means and social connections powered a widening class system and consumer revolution in a culture that increasingly defined people by what they looked like and what they owned.

This was the shift that dentistry in general, and the tooth transplant in particular, needed in order to become popular.[37] Where our bodies became the canvases of our individuality, there was the prospect to improve oneself, to prettify one's anatomical assets. Instructive essays and pamphlets found their way into the hands of impressionable young girls and women, urging them to take particular care of their teeth above all else. 'Unpowdered curls', Mayer Lewis opined, were forgivable for a busy lady but 'no excuse can be made, or taken for a dirty and foul set of teeth'.[38] Poetry and literature, too, reflected the new importance of teeth. 'Take, gentle Creatures, take a Friend's Advice', wrote the poet John Breval, 'in polishing your Teeth be wond'rous nice.' His message could grace a poster in any modern dental waiting room: brush twice a day, and don't eat too much sugar or your teeth will decay and your breath stink (though he also added the threat that a woman with a noxious mouth would never get a husband).[39]

The professional dentists taking Fauchard's lead agreed that a healthy, attractive body included a set of white teeth.[40] They offered services for those who wanted to decorate their bodies or hide the marks of time or disease. The dentist Nicholas Dubois de Chemant compared the eyes to the teeth – where the eyes were a window to the soul, the teeth were the index of health. A good set of both were needed, he wrote, to be beautiful (and he happened to provide the latter in artificial form, fashioned from a porcelain paste procured from the enterprising Wedgwood).[41] The Italian-born British dentist Bartholomew Ruspini and his son also prioritized looks. You could make an appointment at their palatial homes to sort out your facial deformities and 'the foetid smell arising from carious Teeth and diseased Gums'.[42]

So-called 'society dentists' like de Chemant and Ruspini attracted the wealthiest and most discerning patients, and accordingly surrounded themselves with the trappings of high society, with high-ceilinged, well-lit surgeries and fashionable accessories and tools. In 1784 Richard Dighton depicted their kind in his painting 'The London Dentist', a companion piece to 'The Country Tooth-Drawer' mentioned earlier, which portrayed their rustic counterparts. It shows a foppish foreign dentist operating from his well-appointed, sumptuous home overlooking St James's Palace. There are no hoof nippers in sight. Instead he has a black servant to hold his specially designed 'dental key', an eighteenth-century instrument specially designed to clamp onto his patient's tooth and lever it out with one quick, clean crack.

With science starting to suggest that body parts might be interchangeable, a widening class system and a growing sense that beautiful teeth were an important part of a beautiful

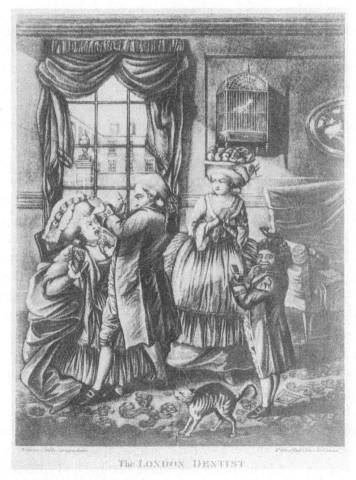

Figure 26 'The London Dentist'.

body, the scene was set for a boom in transplant surgery. It took just one man to connect it all and make the tooth transplant into one of the ugliest fashion trends in history.

The Tooth Transplant Boom

John Hunter was 'the leading surgeon-physiologist of his age', wrote one medical historian.[43] He 'raised surgery from a craft to a science', said another.[44] And for journalist and Hunter biographer Wendy Moore, he represented 'a whole new era of operations' and helped to 'establish the foundations of scientific surgery'.[45] This dour Scottish surgeon with the shock of red hair and famously brusque manner undeniably revolutionized surgery. At the start of his life, barbers would still perform minor operations, but by the time of his death in 1793, his approach had transformed the profession into one based on scientific principles. He joins Harvey as one of the few trailblazers whose ideas became widely accepted in their lifetimes. In Britain, his methods were the basis for nineteenth-century teaching hospitals. In the USA they informed a growing country's system of medical education. And when his student Edward Jenner applied his teacher's principles to his own experiments on inoculation, he created the first vaccine (for smallpox). Hunter's values of empiricism, observation and experimentation are recognizable in today's surgery because they endure as the very foundation of our medical system.

By eighteenth-century standards, though, Hunter did things differently from his fellow medical professionals, as the philosopher David Hume found out in 1776 when he sought his advice about a lump in his abdomen.[46] Hume had consulted physician after physician to find out what was wrong with him. Scores of doctors examined him, all eminent men. They took their histories, worked out complexions and treatments like the good humoralists they were, but they didn't touch him. There was no reason to do so. They *still*, over two hundred years after Vesalius published his *Fabrica*, had more faith in the authority of their ancient Greek predecessors than in what their own bodies could tell them. Out of everyone Hume consulted, only Hunter took the trouble to place his hands directly on the philosopher's midriff to feel the bulging contours of a tumour. He didn't need antique texts to tell him his patient had cancer. The tumour was, as Hume put it in a letter breaking the news to his friend, 'obvious to the Senses, and perceived by the greatest anatomist in Europe'.

Hunter had started to establish this reputation in the 1750s, working under his physician brother, William, at whose school he became a teacher and researcher of anatomy. His classes were so popular that sometimes about a hundred students would squeeze around him to watch him dissect a corpse.[47] William Shippen, the famous American physician, sent his son to study with Hunter during his time working in the anatomy school. When Shippen Jr returned to his native Philadelphia, he put his teacher's hands-on dissection model into practice, establishing the first anatomical lectures in America.[48]

After a decade working with his brother, having already earned a reputation as Britain's premier anatomist and surgeon, Hunter joined the army as a surgeon. During the Seven Years War against France, he operated first from a lurching ship on groaning, screaming, terrified men. After a spell removing musket balls and sawing off limbs, he was ensconced on Belle-Île, off the coast of Brittany and claimed for England at vast human cost, where he fought infections, fevers and contagious diseases. When island life calmed and the life of service quietened, he also took the opportunity to study the local fauna. He was particularly taken by the lizard population, fifty specimens of which he preserved in jars and took home with him (along with a hundred-and-fifty-odd other specimens sloshing around in spirits). The lizards had caught Hunter's eye because, like Trembley's polyps, the normal rules of organic life didn't seem to apply to them. He found he could easily detach their tails simply by pulling at them, and then they grew back. Some even grew *two* tails where they'd originally had one.

Hunter's decision to bottle up those lizards would soon provide him with the inspiration to transplant teeth. The moment came when he was back in Britain. He arrived in April 1763 with no job or hope of patronage to secure a hospital appointment, and to make matters worse he'd also recently fallen out with his brother. Living on army half-pay in notoriously seedy Covent Garden, he went after the financial security dentistry could provide, joining forces with a jolly man called James Spence. Spence was the first tooth drawer in Britain to adopt Fauchard's term 'dentist', a respected man in a disreputable business. Not only did physicians and surgeons still consider themselves above sticking their fingers into an eighteenth-century mouth, a 'dentist' was a foreign concept, good only for, as the *Edinburgh Chronicle* put it in 1759, a 'French puffer'. But Spence excelled in his profession and by 1766 he was named 'operator for the teeth' to George III. Hunter spent day after day in Spence's surgery and worked with him until 1768, not only extracting teeth but also learning how to make gold and lead fillings and how to clean teeth and file them. He also studied the roots of the extracted teeth passing before his eyes, noting that some had single tails, others double. They looked, in fact, like the lizard tails he had corked up in Belle-Île. The reptiles' regenerative properties reminded him of how bones and skin can fix themselves and grow into one another. This mental fidget led him to mount several healing and grafting experiments to see if he could make living matter from other animals, including their teeth, behave like the lizards' tails.

He started with an experiment he described as 'old and well-known' and cut off a cockerel's spur to attach to a fowl's comb, where it was nourished and continued to grow.[49] Robert Hooke had proposed performing the same trick a century earlier as part of a suite of skin-graft experiments at the Royal Society.[50] Even then, transplanting a cockerel's spur to its head was apparently a well-known trick some showmen used to manufacture an exotic animal 'freak' to exhibit in country fairs. Since then it had also been described in scientific terms as a 'graft', in 1746, by Henri-Louis Duhamel at the Académie Royale des Sciences.[51] After his success with the already-established, Hunter extracted a cockerel's testicle and transplanted this into its own belly. And then another cockerel's testicle into a hen's belly. To check whether these grafts had taken, he injected dye into the blood vessels after he'd slaughtered the animal – a technique he invented. If blood flow had been established between the two parts, he reasoned, the graft would have taken. As it happened, both grafts did take, though the last one was a stroke of luck – the cockerel and hen were probably inbred, and therefore genetically similar.[52]

Emboldened by his transplants on cockerels and whatever other unrecorded animals he managed to get his hands on, Hunter moved on to humans.[53] For his first experiment involving a person, he found a man or boy who 'volunteered' to have a healthy tooth taken out and transplanted to another cockerel's comb. He made a deep wound with his lancet in the thickest part of the comb, then pressed in the tooth, fastening it in place with thread. He let the cockerel peck around for a few months before killing it, then injected it with ink. After soaking its head in some weak acid to soften the tooth, he then cut it into two halves, reporting that 'the external surface of the tooth adhered everywhere to the comb by vessels, similar to the union of a tooth with the gum and sockets'. Like the lizard tails that consumed his attention on Belle-Île, the tooth transplant was a moment when life seemed to move into a body part, even after death had taken it. At least that's what he thought. It hadn't really worked. He'd stuck the tooth into the comb, but the blood supply hadn't been established. Still, he seems to have convinced himself it had worked, adding that he'd tried the experiment 'a great number' of times, but had only succeeded once.

Hunter's transplanted spur, testicle and tooth specimens have a special place for the Royal College of Surgeons and

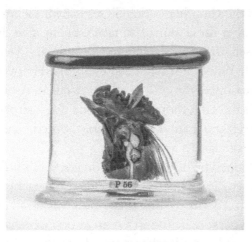

Figure 27 Specimen P56, a human tooth transplanted into a cockerel's comb (detail).

are displayed to this day. They're so proud of the tooth transplant exhibit, specimen P56, they made an image of it into an
embroidered badge to put on their dental gowns.

By the time Hunter did these experiments, enough tooth
transplants had already been performed to merit coverage in
a peculiarly eighteenth-century kind of literature called the
'it' narrative.[54] 'It' narratives – something we don't hear much
about any more – were stories that followed the adventures
of an inanimate object. This could be a teacup, a banknote,
a reading desk, or even an atom. In one unattributed story
from 1759, *The Sedan*, the reader follows the adventures of a
sedan chair as it carries people around the city. One of its
passengers shows off her transplanted smile, and a little boy
shouts out, 'Aye, I know you, and I know my own tooth too
from all the rest. Give me my tooth! Give me my tooth!' But
he doesn't want it for himself. 'My mother is angry with me
for selling it, and says they are not mine but hers till I go out
'prentice.' And he let them go for half a guinea when he
could have got five.[55]

Such a situation with the rich buying body parts from the
poor would only become more frequent as the century progressed. And now, with scientific 'proof' that tooth transplants
worked, it was Hunter's turn to try his hand at it. He advertised
for 'donors', and poor children flocked to sell their teeth,
grimly aware that they owned something worth money. The
rotten-stumped rich were pampered as they awaited their
new teeth, which Hunter fastened in with silk thread or sea-
weed. With his mind firmly on the physical process itself, he
later reported that the transplants worked because of a 'vital
principle' establishing a connection with the new part, bringing it back to life.

Like the Boerhaavian vitalists who came before him,

Hunter believed life was a *physical* thing, an invisible particle that couldn't be seen or even detected by scientific instruments. But Hunter didn't buy the nervous vitalism of his predecessors. After copious experiments on animals living and dead, he noticed that he could find life even where nerves never existed or had withered away. Nerves could, at best, be responsible for the higher faculties of the mind, but not for life itself. He launched his own search to find the one part of the body responsible for life, taking years to amass and study his vast plant and animal specimen collection. Comparing once-living specimens with one another, he looked for a common denominator, reasoning that this would be the body part he was looking for. The brain was an early candidate. Perhaps life came from the brain, but no: starfish existed without brains, and they were clearly alive. Other creatures lived without hearts, so they were out, too. The only thing common to every living thing was some kind of circulating – or at least distributed – fluid.

Hunter cited the blood-transfusion experiments of the previous century as proof of 'the uniform nature of the blood'. Even though blood had a variety of colours and types, he reasoned it was the *only* thing every human, animal and plant had in common. There must, therefore, be something responsible for life *inside* the blood, and he put a name to it – the *materia vitæ diffusa*.[56] It was as it sounded: a material thing, vital (alive), and diffused throughout the body – as Hunter put it, 'a necessary constituent' of each part. So, if you lose blood, you lose life because life is inside the blood (for this reason, Hunter detested the still-common practice of bloodletting, apart from in special cases, believing that it 'weakens the animal principle and life itself'). But Hunter's living principle was different from others in one very specific and important way: it was found in all blood and therefore was universal. This meant that a transplanted body part didn't have to belong to any body in particular. The healing mechanism could create bridges across bodies of any kind. He'd even shown – or thought he'd shown – how this worked between a human tooth and a cockerel's comb.

Hunter is celebrated today for his empirical values – the kind of approach to medicine that detected Hume's tumour and produced treatments for venereal disease, gunshot wounds and countless other maladies. But it's rare to hear about his 'vital principle'. This is understandable because there is no such thing as a vital principle, and this one physiological misunderstanding is rather overshadowed by the greater achievement of transforming surgery from a craft to a science. But his belief in vitalism was nevertheless behind his conviction that tooth transplants worked, and informed the lectures he composed and delivered on transplantation.

In 1771, in *The Natural History of the Human Teeth*, Hunter even suggested how the body could claim teeth from dead donors. Sometimes, he said, dentists even preferred to select from a box of teeth extracted from corpses because there was a better chance of finding a good fit by sifting through teeth of different shapes and sizes and rattling them around to find one that fitted best. Even though they tended to discolour and stain, he'd seen so-called 'dead teeth' last many years. Another potential source might be teeth plucked directly from the mouths of hanging criminals – a situation portrayed by Francisco Goya in his 1797 painting 'A Caza de Dientes' ('Out Hunting for Teeth'). Wartime could also bring a healthy supply: scavengers would scour battlefields – of the Peninsular War to begin with, and then Waterloo – for good teeth, and pull them out of dead mouths. These

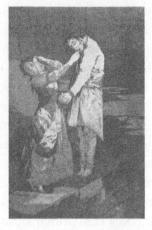

Figure 28 'A Caza de Dientes' ('Out Hunting for Teeth'), Francisco Goya, 1799.

so-called 'Waterloo Teeth' would sit in barrels ready to be shipped for dentures and probably also transplantation.[57]

With the eighteenth century being a society of unequals, however, the widening British class system provided most of the donors. The working classes, or more precisely working-class children, had the teeth but needed the money. They became, along with most things in the eighteenth century, commodities to be bought and sold. Emma Hart – the future Lady Hamilton, wife of Lord Nelson – contemplated sacrificing her teeth to a dentist when she was young, but luckily for her was persuaded otherwise.[58] More people than ever, too, were emerging from poverty as the sharp-elbowed middle classes swelled, and many of them had no compunction about disfiguring a child for the sake of their own smile. The tooth transplants were the first exchanges of body parts to become heartless financial transactions. In the 1770s and 1780s, tooth transplants expanded exponentially around

London but also the rest of the country, as dentists added it to their repertoire of operations. One female dentist in York promised to transplant teeth 'without putting both patients to any anguish'.[59] The procedure even reached the USA. We find it advertised in New York by the dentist Jean-Pierre Le Mayeur, who moved there from Great Portland Street in London.[60]

At the very height of the tooth transplant boom, in 1787, Matthew Boulton – the manufacturer who worked with James Watt on his steam engine – arranged a tooth transplant for his daughter, Anne, his 'fair maid of the mill', who was plagued by toothache in one of her incisors.[61] She was nineteen and was already looking for a husband in her orthopaedic shoes when she felt the ecstatic pain shoot through the decaying stump in her jaw and cried to her father to make it stop. There was nothing for it – the tooth had to come out. It wouldn't be the first extraction for poor Anne, since her penchant for sugar had caused several others to decay before now. But this one was smack in the middle of her smile. Losing such a tooth was, as her father wrote in a letter to his banker and friend William Matthews, 'a matter of great consequence to a young woman'. It would surely affect her chances of finding a suitor.

Luckily, Boulton knew exactly who to turn to and sent Anne to see an old family friend, Charles Dumergue. 'Daddy Dumergue', as Boulton called him, looked after the royal teeth as well as those of the Boultons. Daddy assured 'Pappa Boulton' he could remove the tooth yet retain the smile by using the popular technique of transplanting teeth – something he did all the time in his fashionable London surgery. So, Anne was sent to Daddy Dumergue's place, cradling her jaw all the way from Birmingham. Inside, she found herself sitting side by side with an impecunious fourteen-year-old girl. Nobody bothered to record the 'donor' girl's name or anything about her – she was simply the grower of a replacement tooth that hadn't decayed as badly because she couldn't afford to eat the sugar that was a large part of Anne's diet. Working quickly, Dumergue pulled out Anne's troublesome front tooth and discarded it. He then quickly yanked out the poor girl's healthy tooth – probably with a bit of the gum still attached – stuck it into the gap in Anne's mouth and tied it in place. The anonymous girl would have been sent on her miserable way clutching a coin. Perhaps she lost more than one tooth – and gained more than one coin – if the first didn't fit.

Tooth transplants were so popular by the year of Anne's transplant, 1787, that we don't even have to imagine the scene

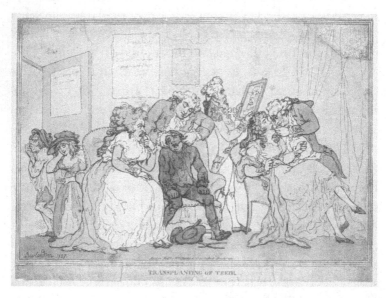

Figure 29 'Transplanting of Teeth' by Thomas Rowlandson, 1787.

because it was painted by the satirist Thomas Rowlandson, who felt moved to draw a cartoon called 'Transplanting of Teeth'. He painted a chimney sweep in the chair, and an old harridan sniffing salts in expectation of receiving her new tooth. The caricatured dentist in this drawing is supposed to be none other than Dumergue's colleague Bartholomew Ruspini. In Rowlandson's depiction, Ruspini is shown working from his private premises in Piccadilly, where he'd been since 1766.[62]

To get the donor's side of the story, we have to rely on the literature and satire of the period. Another 'it' narrative from 1782 followed a coin, a rupee, that witnessed the aftermath of a tooth transplant. Unlike the sedan chair, the rupee's owners are more elaborate in their damnation. The scene is a vignette about a chimney sweep complaining about having to donate his 'property' to a 'rich lady'. The rupee speaks:

> The last of my master's customers was a chimney sweep about twelve years of age, who bought some little necessaries with the profits of the day.
>
> My master, observing that he had no teeth in the fore part of his jaws, asked the boy by what accident he had lost them: 'By no accident,' replied the sweep, 'my mother sold them when I was young, to a dentist who transplanted them into the head of an old lady of quality. But I had the pleasure of hearing since, that her gums, rotten with disease and sweetmeats, did not long retain my property, for they fell down her throat, one night, when she was asleep, and she never once awakened since that time.'[63]

One circulating bit of currency – the coin – hears and relays the fate of another bit of circulating currency – the tooth. But there is a moral tone, too. The 'master' in this scene is a pawnbroker – a figure who makes his money from the misfortune of others. The exploitation of the poor was rife in the eighteenth century, but tooth transplantation was so reprehensible that even the pawnbroker thinks the dentist evil. 'I would rather beg in the streets', the rupee's master says, 'than ride in a coach by such means as these.' Forcing people to sell body parts was, for many, a moral red line then, just as it is today.

Buying teeth for transplant was also something 'new money' did. In a 1773 play called *The Pantheonites* by the Irish writer Francis Gentleman, a lottery winner called Mrs Drugger decides she wants two new teeth 'putting in'. The dentist comes in 'von hour', but Mrs Drugger doesn't like the fact that he's bringing a 'leetel chimney sweep' and her servant has to explain to her that 'tho' he be black, has very white a toots' and the dentist will 'take dem out of his mout, and put dem piping hot into your mout'. Being from new money, she has to be assured that this is 'the quality way' before she forks out ten guineas for the two teeth. 'Cheap as dirt', Mrs Drugger says. 'If I like them I'll buy every tooth in his head, and give him mine into the bargain.'[64]

The tooth transplant reflected the new society that Anne Boulton's father helped bring about, from the obsession with low-value tat like buttons and buckles right through to silver, ormolu and Blue John. The pirate-cum-physician Henri Martinière had worried about this unfairness in relation to transfusion a century earlier, but it was in eighteenth-century dentistry when the poor really did, at least for a short time, become repositories of parts for the rich.

You could see Anne as a Mrs Drugger character – Daddy's money is not so far removed from a lottery win, especially when Daddy is a hardware man. But perhaps we shouldn't judge the purchasers of tooth transplants or the dentists so harshly. Despite his willingness to buy a young girl's tooth, Matthew Boulton is now remembered as vociferous in his opposition to slavery and honoured for conscientiously looking after his factory workers into their old age. And when you read letters between Anne Boulton and her father, she comes across as such a sweet, if sheltered, girl. The tragedy of her life is that the teeth didn't help – she never married after all. Instead, when her father died in 1809, she ended up effectively a housekeeper to her feckless brother and his wife.

The Last Tooth Transplants and the Legacy of Vitalism

As the barbaric nature of the operation became clear, especially towards the end of the century, more and more people spoke out against tooth transplants. The dentist Thomas Berdmore was early to protest in 1766, calling it dangerous and expensive. James Spence added his dissenting voice in the same year. Even where the procedure was particularly popular, the transplanted teeth seemed to cause problems.[65] In the winter of 1785, the American dentist John Le Mayeur transplanted, he said, 170 teeth in Philadelphia alone, though another local dentist claimed to have removed fifty of them, and that they came out easily, with just a pinch of thumb and forefinger. George Washington, who got wind of Le Mayeur's transplants, even made inquiries for the treatment of his own notoriously troublesome teeth. It may have been the increasingly foul reputation of transplantations that decided Washington against them in the end, and instead to have the dentist John Greenwood make his famous dentures.[66]

The plight of the poor and desperate also tugged at the heartstrings. A story in the *New York Daily Advertiser* from

28 January 1789 told of a young girl visiting the dentist in a particularly harsh winter a few years previously. She was supporting her parents and had run out of money and couldn't feed them or heat her home, but she came across an advert from a dentist who offered three guineas for each tooth, and she decided to donate. On her arrival, the newspaper clipping tells us, she told her story but burst into tears at the prospect of the sacrifice she was about to make. 'Affected by her tears', the dentist refused to take her teeth and gave her ten guineas instead.

Tooth transplants had obviously been brutal for the unfortunate children and mostly ineffective for the recipients, but opposition to them increased only when it became clear there was also a danger to the well-to-do purchasers. In one case published in the *Medical Transactions* by the vice-president of the Royal Society, Sir William Watson, the recipient of a tooth died.[67] In 1771 William Cullen – the man who would later propose to revive drowned people by animating their vital principle – reported that, although the donor 'had all the appearance of a sound person', the recipient had still contracted syphilis. Perhaps the most damning criticism came from William Rae in 1780. Rae was one of Hunter's former pupils, who had once supported the tooth transplant:

> A young lady from Southampton came to town to have a tooth transplanted, and being anxious to have a proper one got and perfectly free of any infection, the subject [donor] was examined by some eminent surgeons who pronounced it very safe: the operation was soon performed, and she was soon affected with the venereal disease, which destroyed all that side of her face, and she very shortly died.[68]

Rae's opposition was all the more damning to transplant-ation because Hunter himself, who had clearly since been shaken by the savagery he'd helped unleash, had suggested he talk about the immorality of the operation.

By the early nineteenth century, England in particular seems to have earned a reputation for casual cruelty towards its poor. A German dental textbook decried the 'English trafficking in the teeth of living persons'. Germans did trans-plant teeth, however, but they apparently took them from a sterilized stock extracted from 'young and healthy subjects who have died by violence'.[69] Johann Jacob Joseph Serre in 1803 noted the dangers of transmitting syphilis (something Hunter had also noticed in six of his patients).[70] Also in 1803 another pupil of Hunter, Joseph Fox, wrote that the oper-ation involved 'a defect of the moral principle as one person is injured and disfigured in order to contribute to the luxury and convenience of another'.[71]

Although the procedure was listed in dental textbooks as late as 1919,[72] the most recent reference to a tooth transplant I've seen was a letter found by the dental historian Malvin E. Ring, which concerned an operation performed in Buf-falo, New York State, in 1837. The dentist's patient was William Henry Seward, Abraham Lincoln's Secretary of State and the man responsible for the USA purchasing Alaska from Russia. After the operation, his gum ached so badly he had to have the tooth removed. The transplant was an anomaly – by this time, dentists had realized that tooth transplants seldom worked, and dentures, once upon a time made of animal bone, were becoming more convincing and comfortable with the advent of porcelain.[73] By the early nineteenth century dentists had effectively abandoned tooth transplants.

Although tooth transplants were now taboo, the mechanism that scientists thought made them work was still thriving. The idea of a vital principle in the blood became central to the resurrection of skin grafting and blood transfusion. Skin grafts in Britain, Italy and Germany were revived after the British 'discovered' the ancient Indian technique, still in use by the bricklayer caste. An article in the *Gentleman's Magazine* related the procedure almost exactly as it was described in the ancient Sushruta Samhita.[74] The report was spread far and wide and inspired an Italian surgeon, Giuseppe Baronio, a great admirer of Hunter and protégé of regeneration expert Lazzaro Spallanzani. In 1808 Baronio became the first to perform an autogenous skin graft, lifting skin from one side of a ram's body and transplanting it onto the other. To 'increase the vitality' of the graft, he'd encourage blood to come to the surface by whipping the skin. He also found that the longer the skin had been detached, the longer it took to reattach and that grafts between different animals always failed. But under the right conditions, where the life-giving blood remained, the transplants consistently worked.[75] A British surgeon with strong links with vitalism, Joseph Carpue, also revived both the Indian and Italian methods in his 1816 book, *On Restoring a Lost Nose*.[76]

Debate around the nature of life intensified, too. Carpue himself had been involved with Giovanni Aldini, the nephew of Luigi Galvani (best remembered for making dead frogs' legs twitch by giving them an electric shock). The two vitalists used electricity to similarly 'galvanize' the muscles of recently hanged George Forster, a man found guilty of murdering his wife and child. As the electric shock stiffened his lifeless frame, Forster's eyes opened, his right hand clenched and his legs jiggled in a temporary reanimation of his body.[77]

Two of Hunter's students also publicly and fiercely debated the nature of the vital principle.[78] On one side was William Lawrence (celebrated as the man responsible for introducing the word 'biologist' to the English language). On the other was John Abernethy (celebrated as the man responsible for introducing the Abernethy digestive biscuit to Scottish cuisine). While Abernethy argued that life was 'superadded' to the body – a view compatible with his Christian faith – Lawrence was a vocal supporter of the hypothesis that life was a physical mechanism. Both positions stemmed directly from Hunter's work on the 'vital principle'. One of Lawrence's patients, Mary Shelley, consulted him about his views on this subject, asking him whether he thought it would be possible to create and animate a monster out of body parts. Historians have speculated that Lawrence probably passed on some details of Carpue's plastic surgery as an example of how such parts might be infused with life.[79] In any case, vitalism captured Shelley's imagination. When in 1818 her creation, Dr Frankenstein, assembled a monster out of odds and ends of the slaughterhouse, it's no coincidence the chimera was stirred to life with a 'vital spark'.

In the same year that Shelley published her masterpiece, James Blundell – an *accoucheur* (otherwise known as a 'man-midwife') – suggested transfusion could be used to replenish a patient's strength and save his or her life. Blundell would be called upon again and again to attend helpless young women dying in dank, Regency living rooms for want of blood, or at least the vital principle he thought was inside. But he could only watch them die.[80] He'd recently read the thesis of a man called John Henry Leacock, a sugar planter's son from Barbados, who went to Edinburgh Medical School and defended a thesis on blood transfusion. In that thesis, he described the situation familiar to Blundell – the woman who 'trembles on the brink of the grave'.[81] His experiments on cats and dogs showed that inter-species transfusion always failed, but the animals often accepted blood from those of the same species. Transfusion ought to work for humans, too, he insisted, but only if human blood was used in human bodies. Blundell set up his own experiments on dogs and came to a similar conclusion, that 'it becomes of the utmost importance, that we should be able to supply, the human vessels with the human blood'. But it wasn't the fluid itself he was hoping to replace – it's not necessary, he said, 'to throw into the vessels as much blood as they have lost'.[82] He was looking for the most vital blood, so used male donors where possible since their larger muscles and greater supply of vessels meant their blood was supposedly more potent.

To increase the likelihood of preserving the blood's vital properties, Blundell invented a couple of devices to help less experienced midwives who struggled to operate a syringe. To these he gave torture-house names: one was

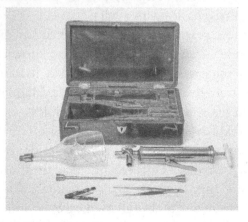

Figure 30 Blundell's Impellor.

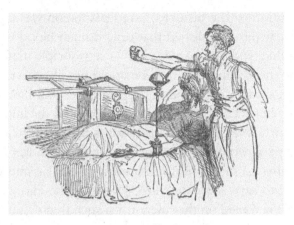

Figure 31 Blundell's Gravitator, as depicted in *The Lancet*, 1829.

called the Impellor (1824), which worked by using a syringe to draw the blood through a maze of passages designed to keep the blood from staying in one place for too long.[83] The other was called the Gravitator (1828), which did a similar job, but relied on gravity instead of a syringe.[84] Blundell preached caution and had a disdain for needless interference in the name of medicine (he once advised midwives to leave their forceps at home: 'Lead yourself not into temptation', he advised; 'if you put your instruments into your pocket, they are very apt to slip out of your pocket and into the uterus'[85]). This prudence he extended to transfusion, recommending that 'in the present state of knowledge, at least, the operation would be justifiable in the most desperate cases only'.[86] When all that remained was to watch a person die, though, they might as well try. It might just save the life of one of these desperate souls.

Despite all his dynamism, Blundell never performed many transfusions – at least, he didn't report many, only ten in total, half of which were successful[87] – but his contribution to the history of transplantation was immense. First, he firmly established that only human blood would be compatible with human bodies – a principle that would become more important than he could possibly have realized as organ transplants came to depend on establishing a compatibility between bodies. It's easy to overlook the importance of this observation because nowadays it seems obvious that human parts would be best suited to human bodies. Second, he was also the first to perform human-to-human transfusions in order to save someone's life. Although the idea of a vital principle is flawed (in that there is no such thing), it nevertheless managed to influence the popularization of the tooth transplant, the revival of the skin graft and the resurrection of blood transfusion. Though it has since been debunked, vitalism nevertheless inspired transplant surgeons to, for the first time, formulate their profession's most noble aim: to preserve human life.

5. Organs, Kidney (1901–1954)

The Death and Birth of Transplant Surgery

Vitalism ran out of steam during the last half of the nineteenth century. After Blundell, transfusion proceeded at a trickle (one survey found that across Britain, Europe and the USA, only thirty-five cases were reported in twenty-seven years[1]). By the 1880s, the practice was effectively (though not entirely) abandoned as scientists began to understand the blood less as a vehicle for life and more as akin to a transport system.[2] Transfusions were nevertheless occasionally successful. But they were hit and miss, and many thought it might be better to substitute blood rather than try to replace it. An early idea was to use milk, but this was soon supplanted by various saline solutions, which promised to be far more reliable lifesavers than blood transfusions had ever been. Some surgeons even reported success infusing water mixed with table salt.[3] As scientists started to see blood in chemical terms, transplantation and transfusion must have once again seemed obsolete – part of a bygone rustic age where human beings likened one another to trees, or a naïve past where spirits, souls and humours had medical meanings.

Unrelenting technological and scientific advances also seemed to leave transplant surgery behind. Each decade, another discovery or realization transformed the way we see and treat our bodies. Anaesthesia in the 1840s, nursing in the 1850s, germ theory in the 1860s, bacteriology and biopsies in the 1870s, virology in the 1880s and X-rays in the 1890s. From antiseptics to vaccination, these highly sophisticated and undeniably effective fields were at odds with the chaos that seemed to accompany transplantation. As the first radios, cars, planes and other hallmarks of twentieth-century life started to emerge from workshops, factories and production lines, the grisly, antiquated business of transplantation was shelved.

Then in 1901 came a revolutionary development from the infant field of immunology that would make blood transfusions far safer and more predictable. Blood typing grew from an increased understanding of bacteria and viruses, of vaccinations and the naturally acquired immunity the body developed against diseases. Karl Landsteiner,[4] a researcher at the Vienna Pathological Institute, had developed an interest in blood serum. In one experiment, he mixed his own blood with that of his colleagues. He found that in some cases the red cells clumped together – but only some cases. He would have expected this reaction from a mixture of animal and human blood – a tendency for animal and human red blood cells to clump together or even burst had been known since 1869 – but here it was happening between two *human* blood samples. Since the adverse reaction wasn't universal, it merited further investigation. Landsteiner thought the reaction must be because on the surface of some red blood cells were antigens – molecular structures recognized by the immune system and capable of triggering an immune response. He was right. After more testing on five of his colleagues, he found two had one antigen (what would come to signify blood group A), two had another antigen (blood group B). The other blood samples didn't seem to clump together at all – they had no antigens. These he initially called group C.

The new discipline of immunology, and Landsteiner's discovery in particular, explained at least in part why blood transfusion had been so hit and miss. In the past, scientists did have an idea about blood types, but they were 'dog', 'cat', 'monkey', 'human' etc., and these were even considered compatible with one another. Now (though his research went unnoticed for a while), not only did each species require the blood of its own species, as Blundell had realized nearly a century earlier, but also there were blood groups *within* species that were incompatible. In 1909 he renamed group C to group O (symbolizing 'zero' – no antigens). He also discovered that, during his 1901 investigation, he'd missed a rarer, fourth group that had *both* antigens, which he added as (AB). This is now the grouping system A, B, AB, O familiar to any blood donor (the '+' and '−' were added in 1939 when Landsteiner and his colleagues identified another antigen they erroneously thought humans shared with Rhesus monkeys).

Blood transfusion and transplant surgery belonged, at the turn of the twentieth century, firmly in the past, and the import of blood typing wasn't immediately obvious. Landsteiner had, however, finally confirmed that some human materials, at least, were compatible with one another, and he'd identified an immunological mechanism that others could study and put to good use. Landsteiner was awarded the Nobel Prize in Physiology or Medicine in 1930 for his revolutionary discovery. His was one of two major advances in 1901 to make organ transplantation a real possibility. The other was arguably even more important and radically altered the way that surgeons viewed the bodies on which they operated. This second breakthrough was the technique of transplanting and sewing together blood vessels using needle and thread.

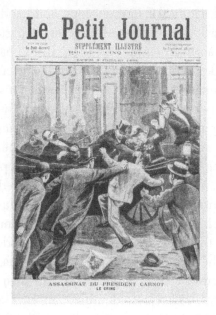

Figure 32 Depiction from *Le Petit Journal*, 2 July 1894, of the assassination of President Sadi Carnot of France.

On 25 June 1894, the French President Marie François Sadi Carnot attended a banquet at the Chamber of Commerce in Lyon.[5] Crowds lined the roads as he went in, and were still there after 9 p.m. when his carriage drew up to collect him. One man present, Sante Geronimo Caserio, had studied the president's itinerary and was blending into the throng, rolled-up newspaper under his arm. He craned his neck to catch a glimpse of Carnot, made careful note of his substantial police escort. A military guard of honour surrounded the president's open-topped landau as he clambered in. Then, moving so quickly Carnot's guards couldn't stop him, Caserio darted out of the crowd, out of anonymity, and slipped past the police. Dropping the newspaper, he revealed a dagger, which he plunged deep into Carnot's back. The president dropped, sinking into his seat, and the carriage set off in search of the best doctors in Lyon, while the unrepentant anarchist was apprehended.

As his carriage clattered towards the town hall, Carnot had lost consciousness, along with much of his blood. When he arrived, local surgeons crowded around him, including Louis Xavier Édouard Léopold Ollier, one of Lyon's best, to whom Carnot had only hours earlier awarded the Légion d'honneur. Stab wounds were treated at the time by identifying and ligating severed blood vessels, tying a suture around them to stop the bleeding. The assassin had severed the president's portal vein, however – the vessel bringing blood from the intestines to the liver – and the panicked surgeons were helpless. With his esteemed colleague, Anton Poncet, Ollier studied the wound and decided to apply an iodine bandage to it, hoping for the best. Like James Blundell watching his birthing patients die in front of him, they watched their patient, their president, bleed out.

In the riotous aftermath, Italian-owned businesses were ransacked and demolished. Mobs gathered to burn down the Italian consulate, too, but were stopped by soldiers and police. The surgical trainee Alexis Carrel was, like his fellow countrymen, appalled by the assassination, but he directed his ire not towards things Italian, rather the impotence of his profession. He presumed to criticize his superiors, which was a remarkably arrogant move, considering he'd graduated as a medical student only a year earlier and was only twelve months into his surgical training. But he knew that surgeons were working on ways to repair blood vessels – Mathieu Jaboulay and Eugène Briau, also at Lyon, had published on the subject, as had the American J. B. Murphy.[6] Carrel believed that, if only Carnot's doctors had possessed the skill, they'd have been able to save the president's life.

In 1901, the same year Karl Landsteiner devised the ABO blood-typing system, Carrel got space in a lab with access to surgical equipment and dogs. He soon found that, even with recent advances in surgery, the thread surgeons used was too thick for tiny blood vessels, which would easily tear. The needles were too bulky, too, especially around the eye, which, as well as causing extra damage, also caused blood to clot around it, putting the delicate veins and arteries in even more danger. If he was going to attempt to sew vessels together, he would need better. With nothing very delicate available at surgical suppliers of the time, Carrel turned to Lyon's famous embroiderers. Thanks to his family connections – his mother owned textile factories[7] – he had good contacts in this area. It was in a local haberdashery he found finer, thinner, 'No. 13 Kirby' needles from Birmingham, UK, and 'Coton d'Alsace, No. 500' for his thread. To help needle and thread slip easily through the vessels, he coated both in paraffin jelly.[8]

Carrel went to embroiderers not only to get his needle and thread but also for the technique. Vessels repaired using existing techniques tended to become infected. If a patient was lucky enough to escape infection, their ageing repair would sometimes bulge and eventually rupture. It was clear Carrel needed to devise a new way of repairing blood vessels, one that took into account their special material qualities. With his mother's tuition, he'd had a head start, and he used his contacts to secure lessons in Lyon's famous textile district, Croix Rousse, known locally as 'the hill that works'.

The woman he went to see was called Marie-Anne Leroudier,[9] one of Lyon's finest embroiderers. Leroudier isn't always mentioned in Carrel's biographies. Even those who

do name her tend to move on to something else by the end
of the paragraph, dismissing her as a 'seamstress' whom he
happened to 'see' and 'be inspired' by.[10] But if you take the
trouble to look up her work, it's unfathomably intricate.
She produced chasubles and fabric crosses with devotional
scenes and embroidered the gold thread that dresses the curtains at the opera house in Paris. She won the gold medal at
the 1885 World Fair in Amsterdam and exhibited some orna-
mented panels in the 'Woman's Building' at the 1893
Columbian Exposition in Chicago.

An embroiderer of such a calibre is an unusual teacher for
a surgeon to seek. Most surgeons at the time learned to sew
from their mothers, sisters and wives. But a surgeon doesn't
need to depict the Last Supper in thread inside a patient's
body, so what exactly did she teach him that he couldn't get
from anywhere else? Fleur Oakes, formerly the Embroiderer
in Residence at the vascular surgery department at St Mary's
Hospital in London, explains what Leroudier would have
been able to impart to Carrel – knowledge that he wouldn't
have been able to pick up elsewhere. This ranged from what
she called 'thread management' (making the thread go where
you want it to go) to ways of working one-handed and ways
of achieving the intricacy required to work on tiny structures
like veins and arteries.

Working on old textiles and working on bodies, Oakes
argues, were similar. Both collapsed and deteriorated over
time under their own weights and tensions. Embroiderers
find it generally more difficult to manipulate older materials,
which are always 'in flux', she says, and they have techniques
for handling fabrics so old and fragile that they're almost
alive. For surgeons like Carrel, his materials are literally alive.
He would have picked up much of Leroudier's intricate

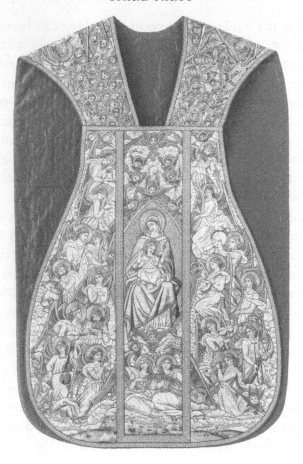

Figure 33 Example of Marie-Anne Leroudier's work.

knowledge of how to handle them – knowledge that is difficult to put into words but is learned hands-on, through
feeling for yourself what an expert has to teach.[11]

Because putting stitches into fine, papery blood vessels
felt different from stitching standard textiles, Carrel practised
using cigarette paper. His busy fingers developed an intricate

way about them, a delicacy unseen in surgery up until this point (but arguably common in the textile district).[12] He could, his biographers are proud to tell us, cram 500 stitches into that tiny space. Through his lessons with Leroudier, he got to know what it felt like to puncture a vessel in just the right way, to know when it was about to tear, buckle, or give way. He knew just how far he could push his materials and how the fabric of the human body would respond to the action of his nimble, sensitive fingers. Thanks to Leroudier's invaluable tuition, he also learned how to pierce only *part* of the blood vessel's wall, minimizing the chance of blood clotting around the suture.

In 1902 he presented his technique at scientific meetings in Lyon and published a paper on his findings.[13] Being able to sew blood vessels together in the way Carrel described would revolutionize trauma surgery. Had his technique been available when the anarchist assassin slashed president Carnot's portal vein, the surgeons attending him would have been able to at least make a good attempt at saving his life (though a wound such as his would still be considered a challenge today). And at the end of his paper, he shared the news that he was using the technique to transplant thyroid, kidney and pancreas, but those experiments were 'not sufficiently advanced to enable us to draw any conclusions'.[14]

Carrel would later go on to modify the technique further and it became the basis for much of vascular surgery, including bypass surgery. Vascular anastomosis – sewing together blood vessels – is the reason that people now see Alexis Carrel as the 'father' not only of vascular surgery, but also of transplant surgery itself. He's therefore the first person mentioned in any historian's timeline of organ transplantation, namechecked in introduction after introduction. One book called

him, unambiguously, the 'first transplant surgeon'.[15] Transplants
existed for centuries before Carrel, of course, but it was the
application of techniques from embroidery – and particularly
the uncredited Marie-Anne Leroudier – that made the internal
organs no longer off limits to aspiring transplant surgeons.

The success of his vascular anastomosis technique didn't
do Carrel's career any immediate favours. Two years after
publishing the technique that would make organ transplantation technically possible, he failed to get a staff position as a
surgeon at Lyon. He'd recently accompanied a train carrying
sick pilgrims to the shrine at Lourdes,[16] where he saw a woman
called Marie, who nursed a distended abdomen and swollen
legs that took up two seats. He measured her heart rate, which
was quick and erratic, and gave her morphine, expecting her
to die before the train stopped at Lourdes. But she made it,
and attendants helped her hobble into the shrine's grotto.
When she emerged a little later, her stomach and legs had
shrunk, and her previously erratic heartbeat was now a steady
80bpm. Carrel couldn't explain what he'd seen, and dispas-
sionately reported it, but was ridiculed by the medical faculty
for believing in religious hocus pocus and attacked by the
Church for not being strong enough in his convictions. He
would be passed over for a position three times before a professor told him not to bother applying a fourth time.

Effectively pushed out of France, he made his way to Chicago, where he continued to work with animals. This was
just as well, since Carrel was not what would be described as
a people person: he wrote off all American surgeons as a
'crowd of imbeciles and villains who corrupt the world of
medicine'.[17] It was in Chicago that he met Charles Guthrie,
with whom he attempted various operations involving
anastomosis, connecting femoral veins to femoral arteries,

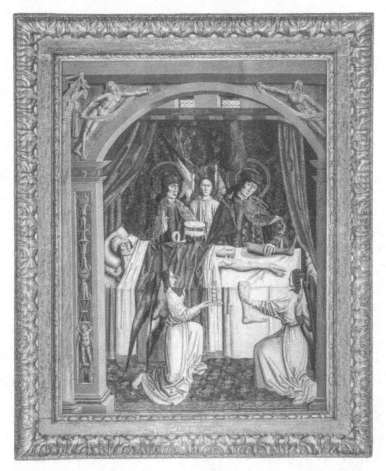

Figure 34 'A Verger's Dream': Saints Cosmas and Damian transplanting the leg of a black gladiator onto a white verger, 1495.

thyroid grafts, and even transplanting kidneys and hearts. One experiment involved removing the heart from one dog and sewing it into the neck of another, where it beat for around two hours. Another involved swapping the legs of a black dog and a white dog.[18]

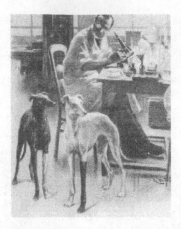

Figure 35 Alexis Carrel with a black dog and a white dog, with legs transplanted.

This latter experiment was a macabre reimagining of a mythical interracial leg transplant carried out by the twins Cosmas and Damian, patron saints of transplant surgery, surgeons in general, and an assortment of other professions including vets and confectioners.[19] Pope Felix built a church in Rome in honour of the holy martyrs. In it was a devoted servant whose leg had been completely consumed by cancer. As he slept, the two saints materialized with their surgical instruments and cut it off. One asked, 'Where can we get flesh to fill in where we cut away the rotted leg?' The other answered that an Ethiopian had just been buried in the cemetery of Saint Peter in Chains. So, the saints stole *his* leg and grafted it in place of the servant's cancerous one. They didn't simply discard the diseased limb, but attached it to the dead Ethiopian back at the cemetery.

When the man awoke, holding a candle to his leg he found no trace of cancer (and he now had a black leg). He jumped for joy and told everyone he met how the saints healed him. People were naturally sceptical but, sure enough, when they marched to the Ethiopian's tomb, they found a cancerous, white leg attached to a lifeless body. There is a clear racist undertone to this story. Given the Ethiopian's lower status the saints could, with a clear conscience, send him to the afterlife one leg down.[20] This is perhaps all the more poignant in relation to Carrel, who would later develop troubling views on race and gender.

All Carrel's experiments inevitably ended in a more or less swift death for the animals involved, though a few subjects lasted slightly longer than the rest. Those, he noticed, were transplants between related animals. All this practice also meant that Carrel and Guthrie modified the technical details of the anastomosis technique to make it more effective and efficient.[21] By September 1906 Carrel had moved away from Chicago and was offered his own labs in the new Rockefeller Center on the banks of the East River in New York City, where he continued removing organs and finding new homes for them.

On 3 March 1908, shortly after moving to New York, Carrel found himself putting vascular anastomosis into action to save a human life, that of new-born Mary Lambert.[22] Baby Mary was born with a rare condition called *melaena neonatorum*. She was bleeding from her nose, anus and mouth. The condition sometimes clears up on its own, but it didn't look like this was going to happen for poor Mary, and there was no known cure. A large sac of blood had collected under her little eyes, and after five days blood was still seeping from all her orifices. Mary was lucky to have Dr Adrian Van Sinderen Lambert as her father – a surgeon at Bellevue Hospital. He'd been up all night sifting through the medical literature, hoping to save his firstborn. A blood transfusion, he concluded, was worth a try.

Carrel had been practising his anastomosis on animals at the nearby Rockefeller Institute. Together with his brother,

Samuel, Lambert sought out Carrel on a Sunday morning. They explained their situation and pleaded with him to try a transfusion by anastomosing father to baby – a direct transfusion of blood by sewing together the two bodies. Back at the Lambert's New York flat, they loosely tied Mary's limp body to an ironing board. Next, they cleared the dining-room table, and Adrian Lambert lay prone on it, extending an arm towards his daughter. Carrel made two incisions. The first was in Adrian Lambert's arm, the other in Mary's leg. He teased out the vessels, and using the technique he'd been practising on all manner of animals, he fastened the two together. Richard Lower had written, back in the 1660s, that transfusion between two animals is simply a matter of 'extending the first animal's circulation', and he did exactly this on two dogs, by connecting their vessels using tubes. Carrel effectively performed the same procedure here, using anastomosis to connect their vessels directly. Father and daughter were joined, his blood flowing directly into his daughter's body. The bleeding stopped. Mary's ashen face started to turn pink. Then elation, a cry – it had worked. Carrel severed the connection when Adrian's brother started to get jittery about her having so much blood she'd burst.

This episode was the first time *melaena neonatorum* had ever been cured. According to Lambert's obituary, it was one of the factors that put a stop to legislative efforts in New York to ban vivisection. And twenty-one years later, Carrel was a guest at Mary's twenty-first birthday party.

By 1912, Carrel's work on transplanting and repairing blood vessels had earned him a Nobel Prize – a prize that should have been shared with Charles Guthrie, but he'd been overlooked by the committee. (Some historians speculate that this was because he had tried to perform a head transplant in 1908.)[23] In his Nobel Lecture, Carrel described the import of vascular anastomosis: 'from a purely surgical point of view the grafting of an organ is possible'. But there was a long way to go before organs could be successfully transplanted. One of the obstacles that had come into view, he explained, was the mysterious tendency for transplants to fail, as if there was some unknown power stopping an organ being accepted by a new host. He'd identified that 'research should be directed toward biological methods designed to prevent the body's reactions against foreign tissue'.[24] He'd arrived at this idea partly because in a neighbouring Rockefeller lab, the biologist James Murphy had observed the body destroying tumour tissues. The body seemed to be 'rejecting' them, and Murphy had implicated lymphocytes (a type of white blood cell) in a little-understood immunity mechanism. He even experimented with radiation and chemicals to keep the destruction in check. Murphy's preliminary findings were well ahead of their time, and Carrel clearly valued them as he spoke about using 'the principles of immunity' as a measure against this biological force. He was on the right track, as it happens, but no more serious research was conducted on lymphocytes for decades.[25]

The ability to connect internal body parts in the way Carrel described was new, even though the idea of connecting body parts to one another was not. Another new thing was how the woman's craft of embroidery came to be applied to the, at the time, almost exclusively male craft of surgery, something for which Marie-Anne Leroudier must be at least partly acknowledged. An embroiderer's skills and techniques enabled surgeons to treat bodies as if they were fabrics, to know them as such, through touch and feel, and to manipulate them with a facility hitherto unknown to the butchering art.

Immortality

After the First World War, Carrel abandoned research into direct organ transplantation, and the infant surgical specialism faltered once more. He still worked at the Rockefeller Institute, but had moved on to other areas of research. Landsteiner, too, had lost interest in tissue groups. During a brief window in the 1920s, transplant science seemed to go back in time to the seventeenth century as charlatans and snake-oil salesmen promised to transplant masculinity and reverse ageing by grafting slices of testicles.

In rural Kansas, the charlatan John Brinkley claimed to be able to fix the 'sexually weak' with a graft of goat gonads.[26] Though he may have claimed they were grafts, they were really just nut-sized pieces of goat testicle tucked under the skin of the scrotum. Aided by his pioneering radio adverts – Brinkley has the distinction of being the first person to 'border blast' radio to the USA from Mexico – he attracted custom from around the world and even had apparent success restoring virility and curing twenty-odd other ailments. The success, of course, was really down to the power of suggestion. He was a familiar and popular face in Kansas, and his patients believed him when he told them they'd be cured (though he would also eventually be exposed as a fraud and sued so heavily he declared bankruptcy and died in penury).

The French surgeon Serge Voronoff also claimed success in 1917 by transplanting testicle tissue from young sheep onto the testicles of old rams.[27] When he wanted to try out this technique on humans, he unsurprisingly found it difficult to find human donors to offer up their testicles to his scalpel. In the early 1920s, though, he turned to apes, claiming that they were a similar species with compatible blood types and that transplants of their testicles could reverse ageing. One British surgeon claimed that testicle grafts could treat senility, while in America another claimed they could reverse homosexuality and all manner of 'sexual perversion'.

While the goat- and monkey-gland charlatans of the 1920s promised a longer life, a couple of serious transplant scientists set their sights on immortality. The first of these was better known to the world as the pioneering airman Charles Lindbergh.[28] On 21 May 1927, an exhausted Lindbergh landed his windowless, single-engined aeroplane on the dust of Le Bourget airfield in Paris. The rickety frame, *The Spirit of St. Louis*, was made from wood, canvas and piano wire, and without a co-pilot or radio 'Lindy' had made it across the tempestuous Atlantic, all the way from New York. A hundred thousand people mobbed him as he pushed himself out of his cockpit after a non-stop thirty-three-and-a-half-hour flight. That week he was paraded along the Champs-Élysées for a million-strong crowd and met the French president and countless other dignitaries. Charles Lindbergh was twenty-five when he made the world's first airborne transatlantic crossing, the flight that 'ushered in the modern world', according to the *New York Times*.

It was back in New York when, after countless more parades, motorcades, speeches and handshakes, Lindbergh fell into thinking about how the human machine was put together. The famously blue-eyed aviator had wooed the daughter of the American ambassador to Mexico during a trip to Mexico City, where he took her up in his plane. They got married in her family's mansion on a fifty-acre estate overlooking the Hudson river, and by the following summer, while waiting for Anne Lindbergh to give birth to their first child, Charles found himself making conversation with the attending anaesthetist, Dr Paluel Flagg.

Flagg had brought along an artificial respirator in case the Lindbergh baby should need to be given air. Thankfully, it wasn't needed, but Lindbergh learned that the anaesthetist had invented the machine himself and begged for a demonstration. Confident that Flagg was his kind of man, Lindbergh told him about his sister-in-law, Elisabeth Morrow, who suffered from a rheumatic fever that had left her heart with a damaged mitral valve. She was only in her mid-twenties, and her doctors – the best the Morrow family, and therefore money, could buy – hadn't a clue how to proceed. The airman confided in the mechanically minded anaesthetist that he couldn't understand the attitude of the doctors, who seemed stumped by what was clearly a simple mechanical problem, a matter of regulating the flow of blood. If something similar happened in one of his aeroplanes, after all, he would have fixed the valve, or if that wasn't possible, he'd replace the entire engine. Surely there was an engineering solution to Elisabeth's problem, too. He thought that, since Flagg had invented a machine to help the mechanical act of breathing, he might be able to help with Elisabeth's heart. It was worth a shot, but Flagg couldn't help. He knew a man who might, though – his old boss at the Rockefeller labs.

At the end of November 1930, Lindbergh parked his car at the Rockefeller Institute for Medical Research in New York City. His appointment was on the top floor of the five-storey brick-and-stone building, with the department head: Alexis Carrel. Carrel had come a long way since his anastomosis days. His labs and surgery rooms spanned the entire floor as well as the attic. He hadn't lost his trademark arrogance, however, and had designed his immense office with his desk at the far end, so when visitors opened the door, they would have to cross an expanse of floor in order to greet him. From his vantage point, Carrel could then study those who came to visit him – how they walked, their gait, the level to which they were cowed and humbled by the self-styled Great Man. Used to being the subject of vast parades, Lindbergh wasn't fazed and plotted a straight line to Carrel, his hand extended.

After an awkward introduction when Carrel held on to Lindbergh's hand and silently scrutinized his physiognomy, the two men went for lunch in the Rockefeller cafeteria. There, over tea and sandwiches, Lindbergh shared with Carrel what he'd told Flagg, pulling a notebook out of his jacket to sketch out what he thought a mechanical solution to his sister-in-law's problem might look like and how he considered her valve might be fixed. The detail in which he'd thought through the problem impressed Carrel. And he did the airman the honour of taking his ideas apart and explaining exactly why they wouldn't work. There was the ever-present threat of clotting and infection, for a start. But more fundamentally you'd need to stop a person's heart in order to work on the organ, and therefore kill them. You couldn't use materials that would damage the organ or the even more delicate blood, either, and such materials didn't yet exist. But Carrel offered to show Lindbergh his own research at Rockefeller, and the pilot accepted.

Carrel escorted his guest to a series of rooms. The first was filled with cats and dogs in cages piled one on top of the other. Many of them had open wounds and were being treated with various chemicals. After Carrel's work on vascular anastomosis, he'd teamed up with the chemist Henry

J. Dakin during the First World War and created an antiseptic dubbed the Carrel–Dakin solution, which was strong enough to kill bacteria but not so caustic that it would damage the healthy tissue. It was another great breakthrough that, a little modified, is still used to treat open wounds to this day. The stacked cages of animals he was now gesturing at with a sweep of his hands were part of this post-anastomosis line of research.

In the next room, Carrel opened a small fridge and pulled out a cat's thyroid. Another area that had interested Carrel after vascular anastomosis had been cell culture and how refrigeration could suspend life in tissues. Moving away from the carpenter/seamstress model of connecting body tissues, his research had progressed to looking at life itself, mainly how it could be maintained in vitro – that is, outside a living organism. He'd found that human parts could be preserved for later grafting, and in an article in 1912 reported that refrigerated skin could be successfully grafted after weeks of storage.

It was in the third room that Carrel showed Lindbergh where this research had led him: his incubation chamber. Steam jets puffed from the wall, keeping his chamber humidified and heated to body temperature. Samples of animal and human tissues were being incubated and grown in around a dozen flasks on a workbench. Keeping mammalian tissues alive outside the body was another of Carrel's world firsts. He showed Lindbergh a sliver of chicken embryo heart, a bit of matter he'd 'kept alive' for eighteen years, since January 1912, in a tissue culture flask. The heart would 'live' for thirty-four years in total. The inverted commas are there because it was later found that, in the fluids that were supposedly washing the slice of heart, were new live cells. Carrel tried, but failed, to remove them and so the embryo would be sustained by new cells each time it was 'washed'. But, as Lindbergh was taking his tour, this chicken heart looked like it might hold the secret to anti-ageing and even immortality.

The final room Carrel and Lindbergh arrived in had black walls, a black floor and a skylight. This was Carrel's specially kitted-out operating theatre, which also had black fixtures and fittings, drapes and surgical gowns. Everything was custom-made in black because of his conviction that too much light impeded thinking, and he felt that black showed dust particles more clearly, which made them easier to see and eliminate. It was here, in this eccentric, experimental operating theatre that Carrel brought all his research together. He'd been attempting to sustain entire body parts, not just scraps of tissue, outside the body by feeding them with nutrient- and oxygen-rich blood or blood substitute (a process known as perfusion). If he could do this, the surgeon could then take the body part out and fix it, then sew it back in again using the techniques he had developed from his embroidery work. He felt someone would invent an artificial heart in the future, too, and this could provide a temporary pump while surgeons worked on the organic heart. A temporary artificial heart combined with perfusion could, Carrel suggested, be the key to fixing Elisabeth Morrow's faulty valve.

Carrel then showed off a small chamber attached to a piston, an early perfusion machine he'd had an engineer build to keep organs alive by propelling blood serum around them and keeping them oxygenated. Lindbergh later wrote that he was 'astounded by the crudeness' of the device Carrel presented. He certainly wouldn't have been surprised if every organ Carrel put into his machine had become contaminated by bacteria. But Lindbergh could see the potential of the

SPARE PARTS

idea, if done properly. 'Suppose we could install artificial hearts and transplant limbs at will,' he wrote. 'Suppose, even, that we could learn to remove one man's head and transfer it to the body of another. How much closer would we have come to solving life's basic mysteries?' Their meeting ended with Lindbergh promising to design a better machine.

After two weeks with a sketchbook and pencil, Lindbergh showed up once more at Carrel's office. He'd brought with him detailed sketches, which so excited Carrel he asked Lindbergh to be his research partner and sent off to have his machine made. The genius of the device was that it had no internal moving parts. In Carrel's earlier machine, the piston was the source of contamination, but in Lindbergh's design the blood serum and oxygen were mixed using a back-and-forth rocking motion, powered by a motor in the machine's base. To test if the machine worked, Carrel inserted a portion of a refrigerated cat's carotid artery into the device's chamber. When over a month later Carrel removed the carotid artery, it was not only still alive but completely free from infection. It was, he wrote, the first time in history a piece of living tissue had been perfused without infection. The chamber was too small to receive anything much larger than the cat's carotid artery, however, and the motor too weak to operate as anything like a pump.

It took a few more years and a few intermediate designs before Lindbergh produced a truly effective version of the machine with a more powerful motor (during which time Elisabeth Morrow contracted pneumonia and died). The design he arrived at, which he demonstrated to an enraptured Carrel, generated enough force to perfuse entire organs by 'pulsing' fluid around them. It used carefully regulated pressure to push a gaseous mixture of oxygen, nitrogen and carbon dioxide through sterile cotton and into a nutrient-rich fluid to oxygenize it. The same pulse, set at a frequency to simulate the beating of a human heart, would propel the nutrient itself through the glass tubes of the device and around the organ, sitting in a bulbous glass chamber. The mechanical process was regulated with air pressure and powered by a small electric motor.

The time came to test Lindbergh's new perfusion pump on 3 April 1935. Lindbergh set up and prepped the pump in Carrel's incubator room before joining Carrel and a constellation of black-gowned technicians upstairs in the operating theatre. Lit by the sun beaming through the skylight, an array of surgical instruments shone on a black cloth, and on the black operating table lay a cat, which Carrel's black-clad team anaesthetized, shaved, drained of blood and covered with a black sheet, leaving only its throat visible. Pinching a scalpel between his thumb and forefinger, Carrel sliced into the cat's neck. Over the next twenty minutes, the surgeon and his team lifted out the cat's thyroid glands, carotid artery and vagus nerve along with their connective tissues. One of his technicians wrapped the right thyroid in cellophane and handed it back to him on a tray. Carrel took this down to his incubator room. Lindbergh followed, leaving the technicians behind.

Once in the incubator room, Lindbergh watched as Carrel uncorked the inlet of the glass organ chamber and slipped the thyroid through. He attached the tiny butterfly-shaped gland to a cannula, coupling it up to the nutrient, then he replaced the rubber cork and sealed the pump. Lindbergh flipped a switch and the electronic motor came to life with a hiss of gas and a slosh of the fluid being pushed through the machine's filtering system, through the cannula and around the disembodied gland. The nutrient had been dyed red, and the two men could see it filling the arteries. If the machine did the job the pilot had designed it to do, the organ would be sustained by the nutrients pumped through it, and it would emerge unharmed and uninfected. The only thing left to do was to wait a few weeks.

And wait Lindbergh did. Day and night, he camped out by his machine for much of the two and a half weeks it took for his research partner to decide the moment had come. Before corking up the cat's right-hand gland into the machine's chamber, Carrel had a technician preserve the left gland, refrigerated in formalin. Now, after two and a half weeks, Carrel retrieved the right, perfused gland and compared the two. Weighing them, it was clear the perfused gland had neither lost nor gained any weight, nor had it shrunk or swollen. The thyroid was infection-free, too, and still produced the growth-regulation hormone thyroxin. Carrel even sliced away tiny samples of tissues from the gland and continued to grow them in tissue-culture flasks. The thyroid was still alive, the experiment a triumph – the first time anyone had ever sustained an entire organ *outside* the body.

Carrel lost little time composing another article, published in *Science* on 21 June 1935, describing the experiment in exhaustive technical detail. Lindbergh followed this up in September with his own report on the machine in the *Journal of Experimental Medicine*. International interest in the promise of immortality was, of course, immense, and Carrel in particular found himself fielding questions from reporters, where he praised Lindbergh and his ability to 'achieve great things . . . in all domains'. To the *New York Times*, he added that 'we don't yet understand the genesis of great men. Perhaps it would be effective to kill off the worst and keep the best, as we do in the breeding of dogs'. These views were echoed in an impressively offensive book he'd just published at the time of the interview called *Man, the Unknown*. In it, Carrel expanded on the importance of 'propagating' the best elements of his 'great race'. Women, he wrote, should be educated not to 'imitate the males' – ironic, considering earlier in his career he'd revolutionized surgery by imitating a great woman embroiderer and lacemaker. The insane and people guilty of 'the worst crimes', he thought, should be sent to the gas chamber. In this book he would, in short, propose doing with human beings what he'd already tried in experiments on mice, and what he would also later try with German shepherd dogs on his private island in the English Channel – weeding out the weak, and bolstering the strong.

Western society was failing, he thought, because it protected the weak, and a eugenics programme should be encouraged to correct this. A kind of high council of experts – mostly physicians – would live in seclusion as the 'immortal brain' of the white race, teaching the rest how to live. A catastrophe would be necessary: 'in order to recover his true visage', Carrel wrote, 'man must shatter his own substance with heavy blows of the hammer'. *Man, the Unknown* was the top-selling nonfiction book in America in 1936, and in its various translations sold over 2 million copies worldwide. For the German edition, he wrote a special paragraph praising that country's efforts 'against the propagation of retarded individuals'. And later, backed by the Vichy government, Carrel actually considered creating his 'Institute of Man'. For his part, Lindbergh showed great sympathy for Nazism. In 1936, he'd be the honoured guest of Hermann Göring, who conversed after dinner with his pet lion sprawled across his lap, and wrote to Carrel that 'some of the things I see here encourage me greatly'.

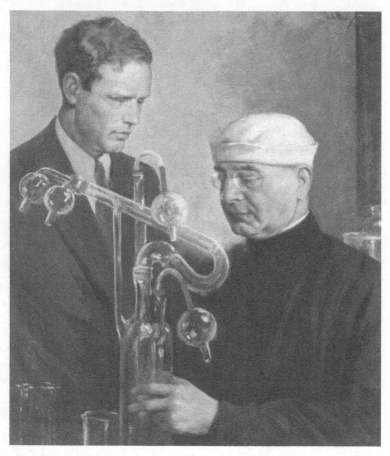

Figure 36 Carrel and Lindbergh with their perfusion device.

In the spring of 1938, Carrel agreed that a reporter from *Time* magazine could come into his laboratory, and the 13 June 1938 edition of the magazine appeared with Carrel and Lindbergh standing either side of the elegant glass machine. Dozens of Lindbergh pumps were manufactured by 1938, and in a speech that year to the American Philosophical

Society, he boasted that he had carried out 900 perfusion experiments which had, collectively, kept organs alive for 100,000 hours, or eleven and a half years. A year later a live perfusion of a dog's thyroid was exhibited at the 1939 World's Fair in New York City. Carrel retired in the same year, returning to France, where he pursued his eugenics agenda. When he was captured by the invading Germans, he was allowed to continue working, earning him the reputation of being a collaborator (though he was never charged as one). The immortality he worked towards did not materialize – he died just a few years later in 1944.

The Lindbergh perfusion pumps had been produced and sold to (or borrowed by) other scientists and doctors hoping to find clinical applications, but their response was decidedly cooler than that of the popular media. Only one scientific paper emerged about the pump, and that was to report a failure to achieve any useful outcome.[29] If the pump had worked the way he described, you would expect scientific literature celebrating the fact. One of Carrel's recent biographers, David Hamilton, went so far as to suggest the possibility that Carrel's claims about the device might have been exaggerated or even fabricated. Despite the silence with which Lindbergh's device was ultimately greeted by the professional community, the idea of perfusing organs gained pace. Later perfusion devices weren't used in pursuit of immortality, but to keep disembodied organs alive while being transported. By the mid-1960s perfusion technology would make it possible for entire human organs to be kept viable for hours at a time, enabling them to be transported over great distances for transplantation. Before perfusion would mature to this degree, however, scientists in Russia and the Netherlands were making another vital step towards organ transplantation: reducing human bodily functions to nuts and bolts, a length of sausage casing and a downed German bomber.

Life Outsourced

The human heart, in many ways, is a simple piece of machinery. The year after Göring hosted Lindbergh, in 1937, a twenty-one-year-old Russian biology student, Vladimir Demikhov, created the first mechanical heart.[30] He had a decidedly mechanical streak, which he had indulged after school by working at a tractor factory. He'd then gone on to study biology under the physiologist Pyotr Nikiforovsky – one of Ivan Pavlov's former students. With Nikiforovsky, he learned about animal physiology and the circulation of blood, and worked on reviving organs, which led him to build the heart. Then, on 24 March the following year, as a fourth-year biology student, he transplanted it into a dog's chest cavity (being considerate enough to knock out the animal with ether first). As elegant as his mechanical heart was, it wasn't self-contained and had to be connected to an electric motor outside the body by a rod, which pierced the dog's chest. It worked, though, and with it Demikhov successfully kept a dog alive, if not particularly responsive, for two and a half hours.

A year later, in 1939, another Russian surgeon, Sergei Brukhonenko,[31] went one step further and allegedly kept a severed dog's head alive with a bypass machine he'd invented in the 1920s. He'd christened it the 'autojektor', and its construction was inspired by two nineteenth-century French experiments.[32] The first was by the neurologist and physiologist Charles-Édouard Brown-Séquard, who in 1857 had attempted to reanimate the head of a decapitated dog. He tried to introduce oxygen into the blood by whipping it, as you might egg whites, injecting this 'oxygenated' blood back into the decapitated dog's brain. The result was what you'd expect. The second was Jean-Baptiste Vincent Laborde, who attempted to repeat Brown-Séquard's experiment on a human subject, a murderer fresh from the guillotine. He'd encountered trouble with a 'stupid law', as he termed it, requiring executed criminals to be passed through the city walls before anyone could claim them, but with a few bribes in the right places, he managed to get a head and tried to reanimate it, though to no avail. Inspired by these two French examples, Brukhonenko decided to hook up his autojektor.

Unlike his predecessors, he could use the medium of film to document the experiment. The autojektor can be seen in *Experiments in the Revival of Organs*,[33] a propaganda piece shot in 1940 for the National Council of American–Soviet Friendship. At one point, the screen fades to a dog's head on a plate being prodded, poked, and even tickled with a feather. It is being kept alive without a body. The disembodied head flinches when a hammer is pounded next to its ear, is dazzled when a stage light is shone in its eyes, and it licks citric acid applied to its lips with a cotton bud. Next up for the autojektor is the revival of an entire dog. As the dog lies anaesthetized on an operating table, the clanking autojektor at its head, scientists drain the dog's blood into a beaker. The shot cuts to a live graph of a heartbeat faltering and eventually stopping when the animal's last gasp for breath is rendered as a final blip on the machine. Ten minutes after death, the autojektor is switched on and the animal's own blood oxygenated and pumped back into its body. Gradually, the dog's heartbeat returns to normal and its breathing slowly returns. The autojektor is switched off once more and the dog's natural organs take over. The film then cuts to show the dog in a cot, weak and unable to move, tended and petted by a nurse as light music plays. After ten to twelve days, the voiceover tells us, the dog is back to normal. Three dogs treated in such a way apparently recovered and, we are informed, 'went on to have families'.

Though it looks quite convincing – I wouldn't recommend you watch if you're squeamish – the Russian video has not been reliably verified. We don't know the extent to which the experiments were successful, and it's possible they may have been staged for the camera, though that isn't to say they never happened.

At roughly the same time, over a thousand miles away in the Netherlands, another young doctor, Willem Kolff, was about to start work on a machine to mimic the kidneys.[34] The story begins in the Dutch city of Groningen in 1938, when Kolff first watched a man die. The man, Jan Bruning, was really no more than a boy, the same age as Demikhov when he first implanted his mechanical heart – twenty-two. His mother was with him as he deteriorated. She was afraid her son might have cancer and was relieved, thanking God, when the kind-eyed Kolff told her he didn't. But he would die, and the doctor knew his death would be harder than any caused by cancer. Bruning's kidneys had failed, which meant he was slowly being poisoned by a build-up of his own body's waste products. Kidneys clean the blood, with around 2,000 litres passing through them each day in a continuous cleansing process that removes up to two litres of waste. But when they fail and the cleaning stops, the body soon starts to shut down. This is what was happening to Jan Bruning, whose blood pressure was soaring, his head thumping. He couldn't even see his mother standing by his bed because his retinas had deteriorated and he was going blind. His entire body itched, too, as it tried to get rid of the urea in any way it could, pushing small crystals of it out through the pores in his skin. Relating this story to his biographer many years later, Kolff remembered feeling powerless, as Blundell did when faced with a haemorrhaging woman. 'I thought if I could just remove . . . as much urea and other products as are normally excreted by the kidneys', he said, 'then this young man could live.' But the young man didn't live. Confronted with this death and encouraged by his professor, Polak Daniels, Kolff resolved to make an artificial kidney.

This mild-mannered Dutchman wasn't the first person to try to clean the blood. Back in 1913, three American doctors, John Jacob Abel, Leonard Rowntree and B. B. Turner, experimented on dogs' blood by passing it through very thin tubes suspended in a saline solution. They formed the tubes from membrane created by spreading collodion solution onto a surface and letting it dry. When the alcohol in the solution evaporated, they were left with a thin membrane. The same trick is performed in theatrical make-up, where a thin film of collodion is applied to the skin, which wrinkles up as it dries into the membrane, simulating old age. The three doctors rolled their collodion membrane up into tubes and suspended them in a saline bath. When they passed the dog's blood through these tubes, they noticed the waste from the dog's blood passing into the bath. The trio of doctors never developed their process any further, since blood also clotted as soon as it entered their apparatus. They used an anticoagulant, but it was a primitive one, hirudin – a chemical extracted from leeches. Though hirudin worked well enough on dogs, it caused heart and lung damage in humans.

Three weeks after Jan Bruning's death, Kolff had a chance meeting in Groningen with Robert Brinkman, a professor of biochemistry. They talked about the properties of cellulose hydrate (cellophane) – an artificial sausage skin. It had other applications, too, and Brinkman himself had used it commercially in another life to purify fruit juices. When it was placed as a barrier between two fluids with different chemical concentrations, the smaller molecules from one side – of urea, for example – could pass through the membrane to the other, leaving in place everything too large to pass through, such as blood.

Kolff put his own blood through the same process Brinkman applied to fruit juices, first adding 400mg of urea to simulate the blood of a patient in kidney failure. He poured this into a 50cm length of cellophane sausage skin and tied it off into a liquid blood sausage. Laying this onto a wooden board submerged in a bath of hot water, he set up a sewing-machine motor to rock the bath back and forth and slosh the water around. For five minutes he had his blood splashing in the sausage skin, exposing it to as much of the cellophane surface as he could. He hoped that the process would remove some of the urea from the blood, but the experiment was more successful than he'd dared to dream. Nearly all the urea had passed into the bath. The sausage casing had acted as a valve through which only the pollutants and toxins passed.

Kolff quickly engaged his engineer's mind and calculated that if he passed blood through a sausage case that was twenty times as long as the one in his experiment, it could be effectively added to a patient's circulatory system. This way, the sausage skin could replace the kidney. He just had to find a way for the blood to make contact with the cellophane, a way to avoid clots, and a way to get the blood through this filtration system in a circular transit, back to the patient. He also had to make sure that not too much blood was taken out of a body at one time or the patient would go into shock. It was a mechanical problem, and quite a complex one, but, given the early encouragement of his professor and these successful experiments, Kolff was convinced that nothing would stop him finding a mechanical solution.

Then, on 10 May 1940, Germany invaded the Netherlands. Kolff and his wife, Janke, had left their two-year-old son, Jack, with a maid in Groningen and taken the train to The Hague for Janke's grandfather's funeral. They took the last train of the night and in the morning woke up to the savage thud of bombs and the spit of machine-gun fire. Kolff climbed with his wife, then pregnant with their second child, to the roof of her grandfather's house. From there, they watched the invasion of their country unfold around them. Pamphlets dropped from the sky, warning of the futility of resistance, and when the bullets whistled past their heads, hitting the chimney behind them, they clambered back down into the house.

While Janke attended her grandfather's funeral – a brisk affair, considering all moving vehicles were being shot at – Kolff reported to the largest hospital in The Hague. It was his duty, he felt, to offer up his services, so he drove there, past the smouldering frames of recently downed aeroplanes and wrecked gliders. Finding the hospital had no blood bank, he offered to set one up. It would be the first in Europe, the third in the world, after those at Leningrad Hospital in 1932 and Chicago's Cook County Hospital in 1937. He would later confess that he didn't know how blood banks were supposed to work, so he set his up like a money bank. Doctors from one hospital could deposit blood or withdraw blood, creating credit or debit. They could even write a cheque to exchange a bottle of blood, which would create a kind of blood debt that could be cleared by donating blood to the bank in the future. This system, Kolff said later, worked 'very nicely', and gave him confidence in handling blood, which he was going to need if he intended to clean it. For this work, he was later awarded the silver Landsteiner medal by the Red Cross, and the blood bank he established is still in operation. But his mechanical kidney was going to have to wait.

Across the sea in England, a little later that year, the Battle of Britain became the catalyst for another scientific breakthrough that would eventually prove pivotal to organ transplantation. Peter Medawar was lazing in his Oxford garden one Sunday, with his wife and daughter, enjoying the peace and the greenery.[35] Then, above the roof of a nearby house, a twin-engined bomber broke the tranquillity. It seemed to be in trouble and flying low over the houses. The family assumed Oxford was the target of a daylight raid so bundled themselves and their daughter into their air-raid shelter. As they retreated, they heard the plane hit the ground in a neighbour's garden and explode 'with a fearful WUMP', as Medawar put it. It was a British plane, and the young pilot was taken to Radcliffe Infirmary, with 60 per cent of his body covered in third-degree burns.

Medawar, a zoologist at Oxford University, was soon called to visit the pilot in hospital 'and have some bright ideas as to how he might be treated'. Though Medawar wasn't a doctor, he'd recently become interested in tissue culture (the growth of cells outside the body). Since the Zoology Department didn't have the appropriate equipment to support his study, he'd been working at Sir William Dunn's School of Pathology, where he applied various antibiotics to cultured tissues to investigate their effectiveness and relative toxicity. He was testing these antibiotics for their effectiveness when applied to burn wounds. Profound burns removing the top few layers of skin, such as those the crashed pilot had to endure, were becoming increasingly problematic as the war progressed. The issue wasn't that these kinds of wounds were novel, rather that blood transfusions along with new drugs meant more victims were surviving the loss of blood and infections that would previously have killed them. Medawar was studying antibacterial substances to be used on the raw, granulated tissue that remained in place of skin, and he had found a non-toxic one – sulfadiazine. Consulting Medawar was thus a sensible call.

Skin grafts were the obvious solution for the pilot, but Medawar knew that grafts taken from another body would be rejected, unless the donor happened to be the recipient's twin. With so little skin left on the pilot's body, Medawar turned to tissue culture and attempted to use what remained to grow some more. He visited Rooksdown House, an insane asylum converted to a hospital to treat war wounds, and gathered scraps of skin left over from plastic surgery operations to see if he could grow them in the lab. He incubated the skin in a trypsin solution – which was known to speed up tissue growth – and found the outermost cells of the skin separated. Starting with a small piece of skin like this, it became possible to harvest the uppermost epidermal cells from it, making what Medawar described as 'a kind of living skin soup'. He had the notion that he might seed the raw area and watch as islands of skin sprang up over his patient. But when he applied it to the burned pilot, nothing happened. He made a second attempt to extend the pilot's available skin by freezing a sample of it and cutting it into slices a tenth of a millimetre thick. The idea was to lay these, slice by slice, over the raw area with a fine paintbrush. They would be more likely to take, he thought, but that didn't work either. Even if either of these grafts had taken, though, it wouldn't have done the patient very much good. He needed the deeper, 'leathery' layer of skin to stop his wounds from weeping fluids and all Medawar was offering was an insubstantial top layer.

Medawar couldn't help the pilot in the end, though he was treated using a technique called a 'postage stamp graft' invented by a Spanish plastic surgeon, Dr P. Gabarró from Barcelona. A piece of skin was cut into stamp-size rectangles which were placed across the body two or three millimetres apart. Since living skin tends towards living skin, the stamps soon grew together and united into a single sheet, the new growth filling the gaps between the 'stamps'.

It was this event that piqued Medawar's interest in homografts – grafts taken from another body, something that had been impossible up until that point. By 1942, he was sent to the Burns Unit of Glasgow Royal Infirmary to study how the body makes distinctions between its own cells and the cells from a foreign body. There he experimented on a patient who had epilepsy and had been badly burned after falling against her gas fire. He took tiny pieces of her own skin (an autograft), and tiny pieces of a stranger's skin (a homograft) and grafted them in place. At first, there was no difference between the allograft and the homograft, but after a few days of taking samples back to his lab bench and examining them under a microscope, Medawar noticed that the white blood corpuscles – the lymphocytes that James Murphy had latched on to decades ago in that Rockefeller lab adjacent to Carrel's – started to attack and reject the stranger's cells. Her body was interpreting them as intruders. This was an immunological response. The woman's body was treating the stranger's skin like it was a bacterial or viral infection. It had learned its enemy, and when 'reinfected' made immediate moves to destroy it. This idea that the body rejected foreign grafts as it did bacteria and viruses was quickly accepted after Medawar and Tom Gibson wrote it up into a scientific paper in 1943 – 'The Fate of Homografts in Man'. Though it was a single case, it presented scientists with a clear mechanism to study, one that would become important in a few years' time. For the moment, however, there were more technical problems to overcome before this information would help make organ transplantation a reality.

Back in the Netherlands, by August 1940 Willem Kolff was working in the hospital at Kampen, a small port town in the northern province of Overijssel, known for its tobacco industry. Under the most trying conditions of Nazi occupation he was about to cobble together an improved machine and save his first life. Now a member of the Dutch resistance, Kolff administered picric acid to those under threat of being deported. The medicine made the skin yellow in an imperfect imitation of jaundice – imperfect, but convincing enough to pass for liver failure and therefore protect the 'sick' person from forced labour or deportation to a concentration camp. He also put members of the resistance into hospital beds and taught them the symptoms of diseases they could adopt when the Germans came looking for them. For one Polish conscript he injected a drug that made shadows appear on X-rays of his lungs, making it look like he had tuberculosis. All this he did at the risk of being exposed as a resistance member himself. Some hospital workers were Nazis or Nazi sympathizers and might easily have reported what they saw. Even those who came to him for help might have been planted. 'Sometimes I was so tired', Kolff admitted, 'I just went home and cried.'

Under this sort of pressure, Kolff looked after his young family while also setting about making the hospital suitable for the research and development of his artificial kidney. From Groningen, he'd brought with him his tangle of sausage skins and tubes. Under cover of night, he paid a visit to the local enamel works to meet the owner, Hendrik Berk, and his mechanic, E. C. van Dijk. Together, they sketched out an improvement to the kidney, a mechanism whereby the sausage skin would be wrapped around a horizontal rotating steel drum to maximize the contact between the blood, the cellophane membrane and the dialysing fluid into which the urea would pass. To protect the mechanism from the corrosive salt solution, the top part of this drum would sit outside the bath. The owner and his mechanic agreed to build the machine, and have it discreetly delivered to Kolff's office. Kolff then

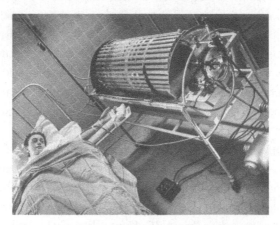

Figure 37 A patient being dialysed on one of Willem Kolff's early artificial kidneys.

visited the local Ford dealership to buy a motor to pump a patient's blood into the sausage skin without leaking. The resultant machine looked eccentric, to say the least: an enamel bath from the local pan manufacturer, a motor from a Ford and a few lengths of sausage skin. And, to top it off, he'd set it in the frame of a shot-down German bomber. This Frankenstein of a machine arrived at Kolff's office in October 1942. A couple of years later, he would publish a paper on the machine in Scandinavian, French and Dutch scientific journals, omitting Germany's until then highly reputable scientific publications so the Germans could never claim his machine as their own.

When the winter of 1942–3 came, Kolff set out to apply his machine to people for the first time. Rather than create a continuous circuit between machine and patient, as modern dialysis machines do, his idea was to take some blood out, clean it and put it back, giving a patient's exhausted kidneys time to recover their natural function. Clotting was a potential problem, as it had been whenever anyone had moved blood around since the seventeenth century, and to bypass this, Kolff at first used a primitive anticoagulant.

His first attempt, Kolff confided to his biographer, was on an elderly Jewish man, Gustav Boele, whose name does not appear in medical records or even Kolff's own papers. Boele was suffering from a prostate tumour, swollen enough to prevent urination. He'd certainly die. Deemed too ill to be deported to a work camp like the rest of his family, he was forgotten by the occupying Germans and officially no longer existed. Kolff, encouraged by his head nurse, decided Boele would be the first kidney dialysis patient. The poor man's arteries were so brittle, the team first had trouble inserting a cannula, so they took only about 50ml blood from a vein in his arm and treated it with the anticoagulant heparin. Kolff turned the machine on, and the drum started to rotate. Next, he fed the blood into the cellophane and it started to pass through the machine, just as he had designed it to. But a red foam soon materialized in the bath. The cellophane tubing was leaking, and the rotating drum was whisking the blood, causing it to create a kind of bloody spume. The foamy fluid had also started to overflow and splash onto the floor. Then the sewing-machine motor that had been powering the drum failed, and Kolff's wife, whom he'd invited to watch this first dialysis attempt, had to step in to turn the drum by hand. After all this, Kolff managed to collect the blood and inject it back into his patient, who died as expected (not that so little cleaned blood would have helped him anyway).

It would be six months before Kolff would try his machine again. This time it was on Janny Schrijver Kolff – no relation – who had become increasingly ill until she collapsed and was taken to the hospital on 16 March 1943. She'd already lost her eyesight and had developed very high blood pressure and a swollen kidney. Now she complained of convulsions in her chest as well. She was confused, and tests revealed a dangerously high level of urea in her blood. Kolff explained to her farmer father that 'Janny's blood is poisoned. We want to take part of the blood out of Janny's body, run it through a machine that will remove the poison and return it to her body.' Having been warned that the procedure might not work, the father agreed Kolff could operate as long as his daughter saw a member of the clergy first.

Kolff took far more blood this time, half a litre, and ran it through his machine. This time, his patient stirred into consciousness. She felt much better, she said, but Kolff thought this was probably due to the power of suggestion and decided to wait and watch. After twenty-four hours, he was at least confident he was doing no harm, so took more blood and again she seemed to be responding. Janny Schrijver was dialysed twelve times in twelve days. Each time Kolff and his team took and cleaned more blood, and her condition appeared to be slowly improving – she was vomiting less, and the blood samples Kolff's assistants were periodically taking looked increasingly promising. Her blood pressure started to fall, and the urea levels were also dropping off. Kolff's artificial kidney was working.

Janny's heart was nevertheless starting to fail, and she succumbed to multiple infections, so Kolff decided to hook her up to the machine directly and try to dialyse her entire bloodstream all at once. These turned into hours-long sessions spent sitting by a whirring, gently splashing machine. Kolff described the experience as 'hypnotic'. After the fourth such dialysis Janny seemed to recover and talked lucidly about her home. After two days of no dialysis, though, her tests showed that her kidneys were still not working. After twenty-six days, the patient ran out of veins and arteries – Kolff had punctured them all in previous dialyses – and Janny died on 4 May 1943, having lived a month longer than she might otherwise have. Her father called on Kolff to thank him for his efforts, and to offer payment, which Kolff at first refused. But, for the sake of the man's pride, he ended up accepting sixty guilders.

Kolff reflected on the mistakes he'd made and wrote them down. Then he ordered a bigger and better machine to be built. The first one he sent off to The Hague, where he had set up the blood bank three years earlier. By this point in the war, aluminium had become scarce, so this second machine was mounted in a wooden frame made by the local wheelwright, and the slats around which the sausage casing was wrapped were made of beech.

Doctors were sending patients to Kolff, but they were almost always beyond help by the time they reached him. Although his machine might not work, they thought, he would at least not harm the patients because they were going to be dead soon anyway. This included one young and portly baker who woke up, asked for a newspaper and seemed to recover. His kidneys even started to produce more and more urine. But then he died, as did fourteen other patients. Nevertheless, the artificial kidney was remarkable at its job, and in fact was more efficient at removing toxins from the blood than an actual kidney, taking out more urine per inch of filtration membrane than its natural counterpart.

On 17 April 1945 two Canadian army officers rowed up the Ijssel river, bringing news that the Netherlands had been liberated. Reportedly, the townsfolk spontaneously sang 'Abide with Me' at the news. That summer, Kolff was sent a new patient for his machine, a sixty-seven-year-old Nazi sympathizer called Sofia Schafstadt. With the Germans defeated, sympathizers had been imprisoned – 150,000 of them. Sofia was amongst the traitors. She, too, seemed near death, with yellow skin, dark brown urine and a gall bladder so inflamed that her doctor could feel it through her skin in his physical examination. Kolff asked for permission to treat her, but her doctor insisted on trying conventional treatments first, giving her sulphonamide drugs and even a cystoscopy to check for physical blockages that might be causing her symptoms. By the time Kolff got to see her, she was incoherent and slipping in and out of a coma. Yet again, these patients were coming to Kolff far too late. And the woman's doctor had even called her family to her bedside, such little faith had he in Kolff's machine.

Fearing it was too late, Kolff's team attached her to the machine anyway. During the first round, Schafstadt started to shake, rattling her bed, and had to be warmed with hot-water bottles. But after a further eleven and a half hours of the artificial kidney's hypnotic whirring and splashing, her urea levels looked normal and she slept through the night. When she woke up, she had clearly improved – 'Now I'm going to divorce my husband!' were her first words. Any improvement was clearly going to be temporary, though, so Kolff asked for the machine to be set up again. But then, without warning, Schafstadt's kidneys started to work. Urine flowed as normal, and she was cured. It was the first time Kolff's machine had undoubtedly saved a life. Schafstadt was kept in hospital after her dialysis and was still there at St Nicholas Eve – a kind of pre-Christmas in early December, characterized by gifts of *pepernoten*, a spiced biscuity treat. Being a traitor to her country, Schafstadt was singularly unpopular in the hospital. It was her kind who were responsible for the horrors the hospital staff had had to deal with day in, day out. She received no gifts that St Nicholas Eve. That is, until Kolff himself appeared bearing one, dressed as Sinterklaas. She might have been a traitor, but she was also a human being like any other, and Kolff's patient.

Schafstadt wrote, 'As long as I live, I'll never forget my gratitude to Dr Kolff. It's only because of him that I am alive and able to write these lines.' She will have remembered him for five more years, before dying of a completely unrelated illness at the age of seventy-two. Kolff had even been able to arrange for her freedom, despite her past as a sympathizer. She had been his first success, after all, and, traitor or not, he didn't want to see her die in a prison camp.

Interchangeable Parts

As the idea that kidney function could be replaced by mechanical means gathered momentum, an American team moved to perform the same dialysis operation with an actual kidney. In 1946 a twenty-nine-year-old housewife was admitted to the Peter Bent Brigham Hospital in Boston, Massachusetts with kidney failure.[36] She'd had a backroom abortion, which had gone wrong. Perhaps the abortionist had neglected to sterilize the equipment, or maybe tried to flush the woman's reproductive tract with tap water that leaked into her bloodstream. Either way, the woman had become infected, many of her red blood cells had destroyed themselves and her kidneys had failed. If she'd been in Kampen, perhaps Willem Kolff would have tried to cleanse her blood with his artificial kidney, relieving the pressure from her real kidneys to give them time to recover, but in the USA there was no such thing as an artificial kidney. The woman's two surgeons, Charles Hufnagel and David Hume, who had been experimenting with kidney transplants on dogs, decided to try connecting a real kidney to her, one having just become available after the death of its original owner.

Putting their patient under local anaesthetic, Hufnagel and Hume grafted the kidney to the woman's arm, connecting it via vein and artery. The kidney itself sat on top of her arm, taped to it and wrapped in moist gauze. They kept it warm by the light of a gooseneck lamp, as urine dripped straight from the ureter into a flask from the laboratory. Unsurprisingly, a few days later the transplanted kidney started to fail. But it had done its job. The woman's own kidneys had kicked back in again just as Sofia Schafstadt's had thanks to Kolff's machine. The woman went home and lived for only three more months, but when her kidneys were examined post-mortem, they looked 'almost normal'. She died not from another kidney failure, but following a transfusion of blood plasma taken from a pool infected by hepatitis.

At this time, Kolff's research papers were circulating in the American medical and surgical worlds. A fellow Dutchman, Isadore Snapper, was so impressed by them he invited Kolff to Mount Sinai Hospital in New York, and Kolff donated his wooden artificial kidney to them. For three months Kolff and his wife went from hotel to hospital via night train, touring the States to give lectures. One of these visits was to the Brigham, where Hume and Hufnagel had saved the house-wife's kidney. There, a doctor called Joseph Murray showed great interest in Kolff's kidney, but Kolff had already given away all his own machines. To Murray, he gave the plans so he could have one of his own made. Working with his surgeon colleague Carl Walter, Murray in fact ended up modifying the artificial kidney, and by 1950 they'd treated twenty-six patients with it.

A year later, on the final day of March 1951, David Hume, now chief resident in surgery at the Brigham, turned his scalpel to human kidney transplantation in earnest. A patient elsewhere in the hospital was suffering from cancer and had donated a kidney before the cancer spread to it. Hume took the opportunity to transplant this organ into a thirty-seven-year-old man whose own kidneys were in an advanced state of failure. With no drugs to combat the biological force that Carrel had identified, it was soon rejected, and the patient died after thirty-seven days. This was the first in a series of transplants Hume performed between 1951 and 1954, all of which ended in the patient's death, though some happenstance compatibility between kidney and recipient meant that one or two did gain a few weeks or, in the case of a twenty-six-year-old South American patient – himself a doctor – nearly six bonus months of good-quality life. For this he was thankful, confident that his participation in Hume's transplant experiment 'would help others'.

The problem that Hume had come up against – what we would now call 'rejection' – was about to be explained by Peter Medawar, who a few years earlier had made a breakthrough showing how bodies reacted against foreign grafts. It happened one day in 1948, at the International Congress of Genetics in Stockholm, when Medawar had a conversation that changed the direction of his research. In his autobiography, *Memoir of a Thinking Radish*, Medawar describes meeting Dr Hugh Donald, a New Zealander and Head of the Agricultural Research Council's Animal Breeding Research Organization in Edinburgh. They struck up a conversation about fraternal and identical cattle twins and the difficulty of distinguishing between them. 'My dear fellow,' Medawar said, thinking back to the burned epileptic woman and how she rejected grafts from an unrelated donor, 'in principle the solution is extremely easy: just exchange skin grafts between the twins and see how long they last. If they last indefinitely you can be sure these are identical twins, but if they are thrown off after a week or two, you can classify them with equal certainty as fraternal twins.'

A few months later, Medawar received a letter asking him to perform the graft himself on Donald's 'experimental farm', which happened to be just forty miles from where Medawar was now based in Birmingham. So, he and a fellow scientist packed up their drapes, surgical instruments and anaesthetics and trucked over to the farm to do the grafts.

All the grafts were successful. He hadn't expected this and couldn't explain it. Medawar had already established that non-identical twins would shed grafts from one another, so some of them, at least, should have failed. He repeated the grafts to make sure it wasn't a fluke. Again, they all took.

Scouring the research papers, Medawar and his colleague later came across the work of an American agricultural geneticist called Ray D. Owen, who worked at the University of Wisconsin at Madison. Owen had shown that all cattle twins had the same blood groups. Cattle twins, it turned out, shared a placenta, and before birth the twins shared one another's blood-forming cells. The cows Medawar grafted on the farm must have acquired their immunity to one another before birth, so they were 'tolerant' of one another's blood. Medawar and his colleague got a couple of research papers out of this realization (in 1951 and 1952), and could now explain that the non-identical twin calves accepted the skin grafts because they'd been exposed to each other's cells in utero. Soon after, Medawar and his team managed to successfully reproduce the same biological mechanism in mice by injecting a mouse's foetus with cells from an unrelated mouse. When the mouse was born, it could accept grafts from that unrelated mouse. It had, like the cows, acquired immunity in utero. Medawar called this 'acquired immunological tolerance' and published another paper in 1953.

Though grafts between plants had unproblematically happened for millennia, Medawar's experiments marked the first time that living animal matter had been successfully transplanted from one body to an unrelated one without rejection. Medawar had overcome the 'biological force' that Carrel had noticed sabotaged all his transplants. It wasn't possible to give humans any kind of useful immunity in this way, of

course, because you would need to introduce cells into someone's body before they were born, but his experiments made
the physiological mechanism behind rejection far clearer.
Rejection and acquired immunological tolerance could now
be studied, reducing the overwhelming, inevitable failure of
an organ to a problem that could be grasped and overcome.
Medawar later wrote that by identifying the mechanism
behind rejection, he 'put new heart into the many biologists
and surgeons who were working to make it possible to graft,
for example, kidneys from one person to another'.

Demikhov, the Russian creator of the artificial heart, came
up against this auto-immune response. Since his mechanical
heart, he had also performed the first heart transplant (1946),
first heart-lung transplant (1946), first lung transplant (1947)
and the first liver transplant (1948), all on dogs and pigs.
Then, in the early 1950s, he would create twenty-four two-
headed dogs by transplanting the whole front part, including
legs, of puppies onto fully grown dogs. Demikhov argued
he'd performed a brain transplant, since both heads were living and breathing and responded to stimuli. His colleagues
were sceptical, so in 1959 he invited *Life* magazine to document one of his experiments, which they did under the title
'Russia's Two-Headed Dog'. The two-headed dog they
reported on died after four days, but Demikhov insisted that
previous two-headed dogs had survived for twenty-nine
days. Even so, all the dogs eventually died, killed off by the
auto-immune response that Medawar had identified. Thanks
to Medawar, it was now clear why all these transplants had
been rejected, and why no transplant between unrelated
donors would work, or at least why any compatibility would
be limited and circumstantial.

Transplantation was a different matter between identical

twins, so even without finding a way around the immunological problems Medawar identified, the first kidney transplant between two humans went ahead at the end of 1954. It
was autumn when Richard Herrick came down with a diseased kidney. He was twenty-two years old, had grown up on
a dairy farm in Rutland, Massachusetts, and had joined the
Coast Guard at the start of the Korean War in 1950. He'd
planned to move back to Massachusetts once the war was
over to live with his twin brother, Ronald, but Richard never
made it back home. Instead, he ended up in hospital in Chicago, with Bright's disease, an historical category of kidney
malfunction, and the ailment that brought so many of Kolff's
patients to his artificial kidney. He was incoherent and
thrashed around with convulsions in his hospital bed. His
doctor in Chicago referred him to the United States Public
Health Hospital in Brighton, Massachusetts, so he could at
least be near his family in his final days. But the physician
there, Daniel Miller, knew there was what he called a 'bunch
of fools' working on dialysis and transplantation in the
nearby Brigham, and arranged for Richard to be transferred
there. His twin, Ronald, accompanied him.

One of those 'bunch of fools' was Joseph Murray, the
man to whom Willem Kolff had gifted the blueprints for his
artificial kidney. At the Brigham, conversation turned to
transplantation and the possibility of it taking place between
identical twins. But would Ronald sacrifice one of his kidneys to give his brother a chance to live? To take an organ
from a living human posed quite an ethical quandary. Was it
right to put pressure on the healthy twin to donate a part of
his body, when the outcome for his brother was uncertain?
And since, at the time, it was also unclear whether it was possible to live a normal life with a single kidney, would it be

right to put Ronald in danger? Since Hippocrates, it had been a tenet of medicine and surgery to 'first, do no harm', and surgeons still took an oath to this effect.

But without treatment, Richard would undoubtedly die, and Ronald's kidney seemed to be his brother's only hope. Here was another ethical quandary. If Ronald refused, would he be – or *feel* – responsible for the death of his sibling? Richard recognized this difficulty more than anyone and, lying on what could very easily be his death bed, scribbled a note: 'Get out of here and go home', it read, but Ronald had already made up his mind to, as he described it, take a 'leap of faith'.

The team at the Brigham had to be sure the twins were identical, so took them to the police station to have their fingerprints, thumbprints and even toeprints taken. Murray also performed skin grafts between the twins, as Medawar had with the cattle at the experimental farm in England. When the grafts both took, and looked stable after four weeks, he could be confident they were identical twins. It was the end of December 1954 by the time everything was ready for the transplant. Murray, who had up until now only performed transplants in dogs, sequestered himself in the pathology department in the run-up to the landmark operation, practising his technique on recently dead humans.

On 23 December Ronald Herrick found himself in one operating theatre, Richard Herrick in another. Ronald was up first, as J. Hartwell Harrison – the Brigham's chief of urology – excised his kidney. He lifted the precious tissue out of the twenty-two-year-old Ronald's abdomen, and the honour fell to Francis Moore, the department's chairman, to cup the sacred organ, as he described it, in his hands and take it to Richard's operating theatre, where Murray was waiting to receive it. He'd already chosen and prepared the area where the kidney was to go and had clamped shut the artery and vein. Then, the team lowered in the kidney and, using the techniques described by Alexis Carrel fifty years earlier, Murray performed what was technically a comparatively simple operation to sew it in. After a pause, they released the clamps and the blood flowed into the new kidney. Richard's body claimed his brother's organ as his own, and it turned from a dead grey to living pink in its crimson bed. Murray would have seen the same many times in dogs, but never in a human. And soon after, it started to produce urine. 'Although you may never have developed any affection for urine,' Francis Moore would later write, 'if you or your patients are unable to make any, you come to appreciate it.'

With his brother's kidney inside him, Richard recovered. He fell in love with one of his nurses and they married and had children. Eight years later, though, his kidney disease returned, infecting his new kidney, and Richard died. Ronald's residual kidney had, thankfully, remained free of infection, and served him until his death at the age of seventy-nine. By 1966, twenty-three twins had received kidneys from identical sibling donors.

6. Organs, Heart (1967–)

When Kolff outsourced the function of a kidney to a tangle of sausage skins rotating in an enamel bath, the result was sublime in its ingenuity. It was almost incredible that an essential function of human life could be reduced to every-day components. Like Vaucanson's flute-playing automata, the mechanical solution was even more efficient than its flesh-and-blood counterpart. The kidney had little symbolic meaning in the cultural imagination of the West, so out-sourcing its function to a machine and then transplanting it packed a comparatively small symbolic punch. Kidney trans-plants would save many lives, but transplanting the heart was somehow more troubling: the heart is sacred, a visibly beat-ing instrument of life. It and the closely related lungs, whose inflation and deflation provide the steady rhythm of life, are ceaseless until death. It was one thing to understand on an intellectual level that the heart is a mechanism, and another thing entirely to confront our humanity and identities by treating it as a spare part.

While Murray was transplanting kidneys, Willem Kolff had been developing new ideas, new body parts that he could replace. During his tour of the States in 1948 he and Janke were on a night train between Chicago and Minneapolis. Janke was asleep and Kolff awake, turning over a length of wrinkled sausage casing in his hands.[1] It was the unassuming material responsible for his career, and eventually the sur-vival of countless patients who would otherwise have faced agonizing deaths. He thought back to how, during his experiments with the artificial kidney, the blood making its way through his device changed colour. It was more vivid, as if it had been infused with oxygen. This could be the basis of a new machine, he thought, an artificial lung. 'I have thoughts of building an oxygenator,' he said aloud to his wife, whose response was to reset her head on the pillow with, 'Oh God, not again!'

Back in Kampen after his US tour, Kolff got to work in his laboratory once more. His first attempt was to mimic a machine made by the Swedish scientist Viking Olov Björk, who had rotated twenty stainless-steel plates sitting in a bath of blood to make a primitive oxygenator. These spinning plates would carry the blood through an oxygen-filled chamber, but although it did oxygenate the blood it also damaged the blood itself. Kolff tried to replicate this machine using old Dictaphone discs rather than stainless steel, and then set out to make something less damaging.

Unlike with his kidney machines, it was out of the question to experiment on living human hearts and lungs, so he used cows instead. But he quickly hit a problem: in post-war Kampen, meat was rationed. The entire city was allowed four cows per week to be shared by all citizens. Kolff argued for a fifth that would be sent to him, with a butcher on hand to put the cow out of its misery if things went awry. Keeping with the agricultural theme, for his pump he modified a milking machine, reversing its action so that instead of sucking, it pumped, replicating the action of the heart. When he applied this Dictaphone disc machine to one of Kampen's bonus cows, it lived for fifteen minutes after which, Kolff said, 'it was killed and eaten'.

But Kolff could get no further than this early tinkering in

the Netherlands. The country had been cruelly impoverished by the war, and had also recently lost its colonies, Indonesia being the most recent to achieve independence in 1949. It would be difficult, if not impossible, for Kolff to get research funding with his home country in this desperate state, especially since some of his more conservative colleagues remained sceptical of the value of his artificial kidney. Even after he had successfully treated the Nazi sympathizer Sofia Schafstadt, some of the most prominent kidney specialists were quick to dismiss his ideas, feeling them too practical, and therefore the solution of an engineer rather than a scientist. Isadore Snapper, the professor who had invited Kolff to lecture in the USA in the first place, told him that 'even if you only find a chair to sit on, you should come to America'. Remembering the reception he'd had in the USA, where he was treated like a celebrity, he was easily enticed across the Atlantic.

It turned out that, once he arrived in America, he didn't get much more than a chair to sit on. He couldn't find a university position of any description and settled for a job at the Cleveland Clinic in Ohio, working in the research department under the hypertension expert Irvine Page. In his optimism and collaborative spirit, Kolff told his new boss that, with their combined expertise, they'd make a great team, but Page wasn't interested in collaboration. He paid Kolff about $8,000 per year – even less than he'd been making in Kampen – and, for his first seven years, the Cleveland Clinic didn't allow him a secretary. The American system didn't afford Kolff nearly as much freedom as he had had when he was a big fish in the small pond of Kampen, and for a couple of years he fell into a depression. He didn't even have a licence to practise medicine in the USA so, after introducing the medical world to the artificial kidney, he had to cram for exams like a student. Perhaps the greatest insult he endured was that when senior staff came to choose someone to advise on the deployment of his artificial kidney in the field in the Korean War, Kolff himself was overlooked for the role. Yet when he did the hospital rounds, junior researchers would recognize and attach themselves to him. Even this upset some of the senior doctors, jealous of the attention the immigrant was getting.

Kolff carried out his new experiments in shared labs. At first he was given half a room, the other half occupied by a physicist. In his half, Kolff set up an arrangement that could be used either as a clinical room to dialyse a patient on his artificial kidney or as a laboratory where he would experiment on his heart-lung machine using a small population of dogs. He'd need to clear away the dogs and sterilize the room each time a patient needed to use it, so progress on his new machine was slow, and he lost a lot of data from experiments that had to be abandoned. The physicist seemed to take Kolff's experiments in his stride.

It was in this lab-sharing period that Kolff came up with a machine he called a 'membrane oxygenator', which he based on the same principle as the kidney machine. Rather than bypassing the kidney and engineering a solution to remove waste products, this time his machine would help surgeons bypass the heart and lungs. A cellophane membrane surrounded by oxygen at high pressure would then oxygenate the blood. He developed his first machine to work on dogs. It wasn't powerful enough to outsource the function of an adult human heart. A Dr Soames, however, saw it and asked if he could use it on a baby. Kolff was reticent. His machine was in its very early stages, as far as he was concerned, but the head of cardiovascular surgery was convinced it was worth a go, and told Kolff he'd do the operation himself. Kolff made him a deal. If he could operate on ten dogs in succession, and all of them survived, he would give his blessing for his machine to be used on the baby. Ten dog operations were performed, and all survived. The baby wasn't so lucky and died, but a second and third baby pulled through and went on to live full lives.

Being able to bypass the heart was an important step in making organs sleep for a while, with their functions outsourced so they could be manipulated and operated on, taken out and replaced. Kolff wasn't alone in trying to build such a machine. Jack Gibbon was professor of surgery and director of surgical research at Jefferson Medical College in Philadelphia, and he had been toying with the idea of bypass surgery since the 1930s, in 1934 experimenting on street cats. Clarence Walton Lillehei created a third 'bubble oxygenator' in Minnesota. Although both Gibbon's and Lillehei's machines had their successes, in the end it was Kolff's membrane design that would evolve into general use, and by the end of the 1950s cardiac surgeons were using oxygenators as a matter of course in open-heart surgery.

The Race to Transplant a Human Heart

In December 1955, Christiaan Barnard, a South African surgeon, was drawn to Minnesota by its growing reputation for surgical innovation.[2] The chief of surgery set him to work studying the oesophagus, but he found himself drawn to what was happening next door, where Lillehei was working on his bypass machine. In his autobiography, Barnard describes encountering the machine as 'the first time I witnessed the life of a human being held in a coil of plastic tubes and a whirling pump'. It was, he went on to say, 'the gateway to surgery beyond anything yet known'.[3] As bypass machines replaced the function of hearts and lungs, those organs became accessible for surgeons. Barnard joined Lillehei's team and completed the normally six-year programme in two years, finishing in 1957. The chief of surgery was impressed and offered him a position at Minnesota, but he declined, preferring to move back to South Africa.

Another surgeon working with Lillehei at that time was Norman Shumway. He finished his training at the same time as Barnard. He instead ended up moving to Stanford Medical School in Palo Alto to develop and study hypothermia, cooling down the heart to make bypass safer, and this would lead him to seriously entertain the prospect of transplanting a heart. While at Stanford, Shumway was assigned a resident with an auspicious name in the world of transplant surgery: Richard Lower. Together, they would experiment on dogs, pouring ice over their hearts to see how cold they could make them, and for how long, and still bring them back from the brink of death. By 1958 they could restart a heart after an hour of bypass, and without any heartbeat whatsoever. This was a major breakthrough because with a stopped heart they could now perform even complex procedures on the organ.

The problem with these experiments was that they were such drawn-out affairs and made the two surgeons, as they put it, 'bored as the dickens'. During one of the long periods waiting for a dog to finish its course of bypass, Shumway started to cast around for something to do. 'We can take the heart out and put it in cold saline,' he said, 'and then we can stitch it back in again.' With their relatively primitive needles, this proved rather more difficult than they'd anticipated. So, they got a second dog and transplanted its heart into the first instead. This was easier because they could leave some of the tissue around the excised organ, which made it simpler to sew a new one in. Their fidgeting around while bored led to years researching heart transplants in dogs, which Shumway and Lower ran alongside one of the world's best heart-surgery programmes at Stanford. In those early days when they shared their findings with the medical community, they were considered oddballs. 'When Lower and I presented our first heart transplant results in the dog to a very important Congress', Shumway wrote, 'there was nobody in the room.' Even the chairman had given up, and left the projectionist as the only audience member.[4]

Shumway and Lower had already built up considerable expertise and experience in cardiac surgery by the time Christiaan Barnard was just starting out. Now back at Groote Schuur Hospital in South Africa, Barnard took a special delivery – one of Lillehei's bubble oxygenators. The chief of surgery at Minnesota had sent it as a parting gift, and Barnard practised using it on dogs, rerouting their blood through it so he and his team could get some hands-on practice operating on hearts. Through working on dogs, he would get to know, intimately, what a heart looked and felt like. He'd know its beat and be able to feel his way around its tough fabric. After months of familiarization, they were ready to make their initial attempt at human heart surgery. Their first patient was a fifteen-year-old girl who needed an operation to repair a heart valve. It was a simple operation, but the team hadn't noticed that part-way through the operation, a clamp they'd fixed to her leg's femoral artery had worked its way loose and blood was flowing from it unchecked, rather than through the machine. With the patient almost exsanguinated, the team reapplied the clamp and thankfully the girl managed to recover.

After this, and a few other successes, Barnard started to perform more demanding operations, including implanting prosthetic heart valves that he'd designed and made himself. He stayed with his patients at their bedsides long after the operation, and most survived. Others didn't. But so monomaniacal was the man that he admitted the death of the patient didn't really bother him. What did worry him was how it made him look: 'it is the ego that is hurt', he admitted; 'I'm too good for that.'[5] But it was in these days of familiarization that Barnard started to think along the same lines as Shumway and Lower: that it might be more sensible to replace a defective heart rather than trying to repair it.

Organ rejection was still threatening to scupper all transplants from unrelated donors. By 1958 the only really successful transplants – those after which the patient survived more than a few hours or days – had been between identical twins like Richard and Ronald Herrick. In the fledgling transplant community, however, there was a hint that this might, in the future, change. Peter Medawar gave a lecture about immunological tolerance at Harvard in 1960, which proved so popular that he packed out not only a large amphitheatre, but also three additional amphitheatres that were wired for sound. Scientists, he said, might soon overcome this biological barrier that was putting a stop to so many would-be successful grafts. Early attempts in the 1950s involved whole-body irradiation and administering nitrogen mustard (which is related to mustard gas), but these had proved ultimately unsuccessful.[6] The kidney-transplant pioneer Joseph Murray attempted to use radiation in a few kidney-transplant patients, but though some of them seemed to do well for a short time, the radiation poisoning weakened them too much for them to survive.

One exception was a man with Bright's disease called John Riteris, who was given lower levels of radiation than the others, and his donor was a twin – a *fraternal* twin, which meant the graft wasn't from an identical donor. Riteris lived for twenty-nine years without immunosuppression, dying of complications from unrelated heart surgery. Murray's success was partly down to the work of a British surgeon, Roy Calne.[7] Since the late 1950s and encouraged by Murray, Calne had been experimenting with the drug 6MP (6-Mercaptopurine) and its derivatives. In his autobiography, Calne tells the story of how he demonstrated the effectiveness of one of these 6MP derivatives by turning up at the Brigham with a dog called Lollipop that had survived a kidney transplant and was thriving after being treated with the drug. At the lectern in one of the hospital's auditoriums, as Calne read the dog's case history to a full house, the door opened and Lollipop bounded in and made friends with the professors in the front row.[8]

Murray performed what is considered the first successful kidney transplant with immunosuppressive drugs on 5 April 1962. The patient, Mel Doucette, rejected his new organ, which was from an unrelated person, but early drugs kept the reaction manageable. After nearly two years, the kidney gave out and Doucette underwent a second transplant, giving him another six months of life until hepatitis (either from the organ itself or from related blood transfusions) killed him. Eight years after the transplant between the Herrick twins, with the use of immunosuppressive drugs, the goal of transplanting an organ from a dead donor had been achieved.[9]

Immunosuppression also attracted the attention of cardiac surgeons. For Christiaan Barnard, kidney transplants were a stepping stone towards his ultimate aim of transplanting the heart, and in the autumn of 1966 he'd returned to America, securing a short training sabbatical in Richmond, Virginia, with the kidney-transplant pioneer David Hume. Barnard told Hume that he wanted to start transplanting kidneys in South Africa. (He only ever performed one kidney transplant, but he clearly did a good job – his patient survived for over twenty years.) While at Richmond, Barnard saw Richard Lower – now a resident under Hume – use the new immunosuppressive drugs in an experimental heart transplant between two unrelated dogs. The recipient survived. Lower had, in the last eight months, performed thirty-three canine heart transplants, in fact, and only three had died.[10] The significance of the encounter between Richard Lower and Christiaan Barnard is disputed, accounts of it coloured by the macho rivalries of the men involved. Throughout his life, Barnard maintained that he had had the aim of transplanting hearts from the start. Norman Shumway and Richard Lower, however, both claim that Barnard got the idea from watching the canine transplant in Richmond. Either way, before returning to South Africa, Barnard visited Denver to learn more about immunosuppression and left desperate to be the first heart-transplant surgeon.

The South African wasn't the only one vying for the acclaim, but he was the least experienced. Norman Shumway, Richard Lower and a surgeon in Brooklyn called Adrian Kantrowitz all had more experience operating on hearts and each of them was, in 1967, ready to perform the world's first human heart transplant. Barnard admitted he was surprised that Lower hadn't already won what had quickly become a race.

One of the factors holding back Lower, Shumway and Kantrowitz was the difficulty in getting hold of undamaged organs. Typically, a surgeon would have to wait until the heart had stopped before a person could be declared legally dead – the concept of brain death had not yet been established in the USA. Kantrowitz had just missed out on the opportunity to perform a transplant because his anaesthetist objected at the last minute and insisted the team wait for the donor heart to stop before removing it. By the time everyone could agree the donor was dead, the heart had become unusable and the would-be recipient of the world's first heart transplant expired a couple of weeks later. While the American surgeons had spent many more hours hunched over patients, perfecting their surgical techniques and drugs, Barnard had one advantage: the only thing that was needed to declare death in South Africa was the signature of two doctors willing to agree that someone had expired.

Barnard's chance came on 2 December 1967, when Denise Darvall was driving her family through downtown Cape Town on their way to visit friends. In the back seat of her new car, a green Ford Anglia, was her mother, Myrtle, and father, Edward.[11] In the front seat she had her fourteen-year-old brother, Keith, and they were both singing 'Lara's Theme' from *Doctor Zhivago*, a tune Denise had just taught her brother on the piano. They were on their way to see some friends, and Myrtle wanted to stop to get a special caramel cake from a particular bakery on Main Street. Denise pulled over and disappeared into the shop with her mother.

Edward and Keith stayed in the car. They were due for tea at four and were anxious to get going. Then they heard a sickening screech and thud. Myrtle was lying in the middle of the road, a crumpled body, killed instantly. Denise had been tossed into the air and landed behind the car that hit her – a car driven by a drunk salesman – splitting open her head on its back hubcap. She rolled into the gutter, blood oozing from her nose, mouth and ears. She was still breathing, but only just alive. Edward and Keith charged across the road, where a crowd had already formed, including a doctor from Groote Schuur Hospital, who had to stop Edward from trying to pick up his daughter.

Barnard was at home that Saturday afternoon, with the Ink Spots playing on the turntable as he tried to unwind after a difficult week and an argument with his wife. He'd been at the hospital a lot, worrying about Louis Washkansky, his fifty-three-year-old patient. Washkansky had suffered several heart attacks and survived them all, though it left him with a very weak heart that could barely keep pumping. He had liver and kidney problems, too, but his heart presented the most immediate threat to his life. He'd agreed to be Barnard's first heart recipient – 'there is nothing to think about', he'd said when the surgeon asked him.

Washkansky had already endured one cancelled operation, when a month earlier a young man had fallen off a truck on a nearby farm. According to the chief of cardiology, Val Schrire, there was an abnormality with the boy's heart, so they couldn't use it. Barnard knew the cardiologist wasn't being strictly honest but was rather giving them a medical reason not to go ahead when the real problem was political: the first would-be donor was black. Schrire and Barnard both had an understanding that, in apartheid South Africa, it would be better if the first donor for such a momentous operation was white. They didn't want to be seen to be treating black life as disposable – a charge they understood could fairly be levelled against much of their society. Washkansky, though, was getting progressively sicker and wouldn't last much longer. So when Barnard got the call that another heart was available – a white person's heart, this time, Denise Darvall's heart – he barrelled over to the hospital.

Edward, who had in the course of the day become a broken man, was trying to come to terms with losing his wife and had to be sedated. He was still under the impression that doctors were trying to save his daughter when one of the transplant team, Bertie Bosman, had to tell him that they'd done all they could. Denise's body was still alive, he explained, but she, Denise, had left it. This was cruel news that Edward received, dazed and unblinking. After a moment of stillness, he murmured 'that's pretty hard luck'. And then Bosman pushed on, voice shaking. By giving his consent for the doctors to use his daughter's heart, he could help them save another man's life. In a later interview, Edward said that it took him four minutes to reach his decision. During this time, he thought about the birthday cake she made for him with the words 'Daddy We Love You' iced on top, how with her first pay cheque she had bought him a bathrobe. In the company of these memories he wept bitterly, but also knew what had to be done. 'If you can't save my daughter,' the shattered man told the doctors, 'you must try to save this man.'[12]

In the very early hours of the following day Barnard cut into Washkansky's chest. He'd been put under anaesthetic after leaving instructions for Barnard to tell his wife the operation was 'in the bag'. Barnard described what he saw inside as a 'heaving waste of ruin and a ravaged heart', which was faltering 'like a boxer about to collapse in the ring'. It was hard to believe such a used-up organ could have sustained anyone as long as it had. Barnard made his way to the other operating theatre, through a connecting corridor, to find his brother Marius, who was one of his operating team, waiting for him. They were ready.

At 2.20 a.m. they turned off Denise's ventilator. One of the team, Terry O'Donovan, insisted they couldn't cut into a beating heart. Barnard, urged by his brother, considered overruling O'Donovan. If they waited for the heart to stop naturally, it would be damaged, just as had happened for Adrian Kantrowitz in Brooklyn, and they had a responsibility to their patient. Much later, after Christiaan's death, the writer Donald McRae interviewed Marius Barnard, who admitted that they had potassium injected into the heart to artificially stop it for a short period – a move they agreed at the time to keep secret. When the brothers excised the heart. O'Donovan looked on without a word.

As the group of surgeons working on Denise prepared her heart for excision, Barnard made his way back to Washkansky's operating theatre. His circulatory system had been rerouted, away from his heart and through a bypass machine, which would mechanically suspend his life for a time. After resolving a crisis in which the surgical team nearly killed Washkansky by inadvertently introducing air bubbles into the machinery, Barnard went to collect the heart.

In Denise's operating theatre now, Barnard cut out the petite, almost-blue heart, putting it in a container Marius held out, filled with cold Ringer's solution – sodium, potassium and calcium chlorides dissolved in distilled water. Taking this from his brother, he made his way back to the other theatre, where Washkansky's open chest awaited him. He severed the existing, swollen heart from its moorings, and lifted it out of his body, leaving a veritable chasm of a hole. 'I had never seen a chest without a heart', he wrote later, reflecting on how Washkansky's life was effectively being stored eight feet away from his body, in a machine.

Denise's heart looked tiny and insignificant in such a vast canyon of a chest cavity. By 5.43, the team were ready to restart it in its new body. They sent shockwaves through it, trying to jolt it to life, but it lay paralysed. 'It seemed like hours,' wrote Barnard, but eventually the heart 'began to roll with the lovely rhythm of life' and they switched off the machine. Then the heart faltered and stopped. Washkansky's blood pressure started to drop. The machine was switched back on and the heart beat once more. Five minutes later, they switched the machine off again, and the heart failed again. After one more attempt, at 6.13, Barnard had the machine turned off for a third time. The heart hesitated but decided this time to beat more strongly. And it continued to beat. Barnard watched the heart beat for a while, his eye on the green readout of the EKG machine. The surgeons shook hands over the beating heart of Denise Darvall in the chest of Louis Washkansky.

Outside the operating theatre and with the vein in his neck visibly throbbing, Barnard brought an avocado sandwich to his lips, taking a few hard puffs of his cigarette between bites. Washkansky was on a trolley now, with no fewer than nine drips sprouting out of his body. Some fed it with vital, life-sustaining nutrients, others with equally vital immuno-suppressive poisons. Encasing his trolley was a sterile plastic tent shielding his weakened frame from infection. Within an hour, all over South Africa and the world, phones were ringing with the news of a world first.

Stuffed with a cocktail of immunosuppressive drugs, Washkansky opened his eyes. Over the next two and a half weeks, he improved steadily. An early press photo showed him in his hospital bed staring into the lens, hands folded across his chest. The newspapers also ran with an image of Barnard waving from his speedboat, *Pacemaker*. Barnard's surgical rivals have all since admitted intense disappointment that they weren't the first to transplant a human heart, but Norman Shumway's and Richard Lower's professional wounds were perhaps deepest. They'd done more work than anyone on developing the surgery itself, and when Barnard was interviewed, he'd say only that 'we were all at the same stage in this work. It was a classic case of who got the first set of right circumstances.' Shumway and Barnard didn't get on particularly well when they were both training in Minnesota but had grown to hate one another as their transplant race progressed. The dignified Shumway nevertheless praised Barnard in his interviews, as did Lower, though others spoke out about how Shumway had 'history stolen from him'.[13] It was Washkansky himself who gave Barnard the moniker that seems to have stuck: the man with the golden hands.

Groote Schuur Hospital was crammed with the world's reporters and television crews. Barnard embraced celebrity. His ease with the media and sense of drama resulted in *The Times* reporting that 'tonight I heard the beat of a borrowed heart' and one *New York Daily News* report running with 'Louis Washkansky's boom-de-boom sounded all right to me'. Though journalists couldn't directly interview Washkansky for risk of infection, Barnard had allowed crews to film him from the door, setting up a microphone to amplify the EKG machine. Barnard had arthritis, which made a complicated surgical feat all the more impressive, and he took advantage of the idea that the man the newspapers kept referring to as 'handsome' was also disabled – 'it's no good feeling sorry for myself but I just don't know how long I will be able to go on operating'.[14] They gave Washkansky a boiled egg, and that afternoon an article appeared in the *Cape Argus* proclaiming, 'Heart Man: I'm Hungry'. They gave him chicken and potatoes, and they ran with that as a newsworthy story, too. In their 15 December 1967 issue, *Life* magazine had planned to run with a cover of Audrey Hepburn, but she was bumped by Washkansky.

A body replete with poisons, however, is a weak body, and while he was providing good copy for the press, inside his chest Denise's heart was struggling. After two weeks Washkansky's breathing started to fail, and his chest hurt. He was also running a fever. Barnard and his team looked at Washkansky's notes, but they were in uncharted territory, and all they could do was guess what to do next. His drugs had wiped out his immune system and he'd developed pneumonia in both lungs. Washkansky was back on the heart-lung machine, buying time for Barnard to think what to do next.

It wasn't long before the chief of cardiology called: 'Chris, it's all over.' Barnard gave the order for Washkansky's wife to come to her husband's bedside. It was early morning and silent outside when Ann Washkansky's car pulled into the car park and switched off the engine. She left her fourteen-year-old son in the car. Louis was unresponsive when she walked in. There seemed little point in worrying about infection now, and for the first time in weeks she held her husband in her arms. With the tears flowing, she freely reminisced out loud about their life together. Ann wanted to stay with her husband until the end, but their son was outside in the car, crying alone in the darkness. So, she gave Louis, whom she'd always called her 'Washy', one final, tender kiss, and was supported out of the ward. As Ann and her boy drove through a sleeping city, her husband's EKG machine showed a flat, green line. A nurse started to weep, and it was more than Barnard could bear. He went to the doctors' tearoom and simply stood for a while, then made his way to the balcony, where he watched the sun rise and felt alone. A few hours later, Washkansky's body was on a marble slab. Denise's heart was intact, but blue lungs confirmed that pneumonia had killed the first heart-transplant recipient.

Though hospital representatives, including Barnard's brother, Marius, attended Washkansky's funeral, Barnard himself didn't. He and his wife were being flown first class to the USA, where they'd stay in hotel suites bigger than their entire home in South Africa.

Thanks to a high-profile recent past, many people know at least a little about this chapter in the history of transplant surgery. Most people have heard of Barnard. The transplant he performed on Washkansky was big news at the time, as big as the moon landings would be a year and a half later. Barnard was well known for courting the media, but the heart's symbolic richness must have also helped the headlines. It's the *festejo* dancer of the body – a symbol of energy, life and love. It's the seat of the soul, a feeling organ, an organ you'd sing about, and Barnard had tamed – even dominated – it. Behind closed doors he was reputedly a tyrant, but to his public he exuded glamour, using his fame to, as the *Daily Mail* put it, break hearts as well as heal them. The *Los Angeles Times* reported on his affairs with actresses Gina Lollobrigida and Sophia Loren, and 'an unidentified Miss South Africa'. His dalliances and their media coverage brought a certain star quality to transplantation, and he also represented something of a technical golden age. With his agile yet famously arthritic hands, he'd conquered the traditional 'seat of the soul', proving that even this most emotional and irrational of organs could be considered merely a component in a vastly complicated human machine.

Heart transplants captured the public's imagination far more effectively than kidneys ever could. Roy Calne learned this well after he performed the first kidney transplant in Europe. Journalists arrived at his house in Cambridge to interview him but they immediately lost interest when Calne's wife told them that the first heart transplant in Britain had taken place the same day. They could still make the press conference on time, she added, if they ran to catch the train, so they thanked her and sprinted off to report on the more newsworthy operation. The Etruscans may have associated kidneys with love, but for most of us kidneys, along with livers, are more evocative of wartime food.

Washkansky's operation was quickly followed by four more. Adrian Kantrowitz performed the second tragic transplant in Brooklyn, attempting to save the life of a seventeen-day-old baby with a graft from an anencephalic baby. The baby died within a few hours. A few days after that, on 3 January, Barnard welcomed in the New Year with another heart transplant from a 'mixed blood male' into a fifty-eight-year-old white dentist, Philip Blaiberg. Blaiberg said he wanted to be 'a well man or a dead man',[15] and he lived just over a year and a half, during which time he was pictured swimming, enjoying his new health. A few days after Blaiberg's transplant, Norman Shumway performed *his* first, but the patient survived only two weeks.

More heart transplants followed. A French team performed the first heart transplant in Europe in April 1968. In Sapporo, also in 1968, an eminent professor performed the first in Japan, which was until 1999 the only one to be carried out in that country. After that, more teams throughout the world started to report their national firsts, including in Britain, where the surgeons stood on the steps clad in their surgical gowns as the Queen's Guard paraded by in national celebration, a band playing the national anthem and 'Land of Hope and Glory'. Back in the USA, the renowned surgeon Denton Cooley implanted the first completely artificial heart in 1969, which worked for sixty-four hours until a donor was found, though the new human heart pumped for only thirty-two hours before the recipient died of kidney failure and pneumonia. By the end of 1968, 102 transplants had been performed and by 1970 a further 64.[16]

Though these numbers tell a seemingly successful tale, it was also during this period that organ transplants started to unravel. On 25 May 1968, Richard Lower performed his first transplant, in Richmond. The donor was a fifty-six-year-old, working-class black man, Bruce Tucker, who'd been drinking with friends after his shift at an egg-packing plant. He'd fallen over and split his head open on the pavement. When Tucker's brothers came to claim their sibling's body, it was only then they found his heart and kidneys had been harvested. As well as not bothering to seek consent, Lower had also illegally relied on the diagnosis of brain death. The Tucker family tried to prosecute the surgeon, arguing that the transplant team 'engaged in a systematic and nefarious scheme to use Bruce Tucker's heart and hastened his death by shutting off the mechanical support systems'. In this trial – the first ever to ask a jury to consider brain death – they found Lower not liable for hastening Tucker's death. But it must be said that he had, as the Tuckers' lawyer pointed out, treated Tucker as one of the 'faceless black masses of society'.[17]

The outcomes of most of these transplants also made for miserable reading. Roy Calne, in his autobiography, wrote that the media treated heart transplants with the same enthusiasm they had for the outbreak of war. And these twentieth-century transplants are, in a way, war stories. The surgeons are seen to have *conquered* the body, staking claims to dominance reminiscent of those asserted by earlier generations of anatomists who rushed to describe and name body parts after themselves. Barnard is perhaps still the first person to come to mind when you say the word 'transplant'. The heart transplant has been seen as a race, like the arms race or the space race, and he won it. The operation itself is technically fairly simple – 'any cardiac surgeon can technically transplant a heart', Calne wrote, but it was the management of the drugs and the rest of the infrastructure to take care of the recipient that was lacking. In a devastating sentence, he concluded that 'virtually all these poor patients therefore perished, having satisfied the macho aspirations of their surgeons'.[18] As patient after patient rejected their organs or succumbed to complications arising from the drugs, transplant centres started to close down as quickly as they'd sprouted.

The term 'spare parts' is itself inextricably linked to this specific moment in the mid-twentieth century, and it reflects the 'macho' attitudes Calne recognized in his colleagues. Amongst those surgeons being celebrated on the steps of Harefield Hospital after the UK's first heart transplant was Donald Longmore. He wrote a book about transplant surgery in 1969, calling it *Spare-Part Surgery*. The title captured a certain spirit of modernism and medical progress. With a jigsaw heart on the cover, his book introduced the surgeon as a cross between a super-talented mechanic and daredevil airman. Performing a transplant, he wrote, was like a pilot trying to repair the 'defective engine of a single-engined aircraft halfway over the Atlantic'. Just as the aeronaut had to preserve lift in the air, the surgeon had to maintain life in the patient; just as the engineer needed to keep the fuel flowing, the surgeon had to keep the blood pumping. If either failed, the catastrophe would be absolute – 'there is no question of reassembling the pieces and trying once again'.[19]

Perhaps this is what it felt like at the forefront of transplantation in the 1960s, and it's certainly a term that means 'transplantation' to many people, but very rarely today will you hear a transplant professional referring to 'spare parts'. It is dated for a few reasons. First, it's not as if transplant surgeons have 'spare' hearts and lungs lying around. As organ transplantation has matured, it's become a long, difficult and uncertain pathway to safely and ethically get hold of an organ for a potential recipient. Second, no professional would refer to another person's body in terms of their 'parts', which would be particularly disrespectful to donors – evocative, perhaps, of the seventeenth-century mechanist term 'emittent'. Some of the cases in this book show how, historically, donors have simply been erased from the story, present only through the phantom of their body parts. This was especially true for eighteenth-century tooth transplants, where 'donors' were disposable, low-status, poor and powerless children. Third, it was never the case that transplants were performed by a single genius. Particularly now, they involve a large group both inside the operating theatre and outside, including an immense network of clinical and non-clinical specialists. Longmore might have chosen to depict the surgeon as part of a dance troupe or a Formula 1 pit crew, or an able seaman trying to de-rig a schooner in a storm. He could have emphasized how transplants were team efforts. But instead he chose what any dusty-kneed war-era boy might: a lone, heroic pilot – someone like Biggles. Or perhaps Charles Lindbergh.

For these reasons and more, 'spare-part surgery' is an historical term.

Of those technical challenges emerging as far back as the early nineteenth century, when transplantation could conceivably save lives, rejection had proved a hurdle too high to jump. Since the very first years of the twentieth century it had been possible to sew organs into bodies. Then, rejection was nothing but an unnamed biological force. Shortly after, it became possible to maintain life outside a body, meaning that organs could be given the chance to recover themselves, or even kept alive on their journey from one seat to another. But rejection after rejection, even when the patient had been put on drugs, had meant transplantation had effectively ground to a halt.

Then, in 1977, Roy Calne attended a talk by the Belgian Jean-François Borel at the British Society for Immunology with his immunologist colleague David White.[20] The two men listened as Borel spoke about a drug from the Swiss drug company Sandoz, who had, since the late 1950s, asked employees to collect soil samples whenever they travelled abroad for meetings, and even from their holidays. These samples they'd scrutinize in the lab, where they'd look for fungi with immunosuppressive or anti-cancer properties. Under this programme, they tested about twenty samples per week. At the end of January 1972, sample 24-556, collected by an employee on holiday in Norway, showed great immunosuppressive abilities. Its structure was cyclical, and it was derived from fungal spores, so they called it cyclosporin A.

Calne managed to get a sample of cyclosporin and set up a series of heart transplants between rats. The operations were an unprecedented success, and further experimental transplants involving more rats were similarly encouraging. When he contacted the drug company for more, he was told they'd stopped making it, but he could have what was lying around in the lab. So Calne accepted this gift and used it in yet more successful kidney and heart grafts in dogs and pigs.

He needed more of the drug to try it in a human transplant, so set out for Basel to convince the businessmen at Sandoz that cyclosporin would be a worthwhile investment. The drug company 'reluctantly agreed' to produce the drug for humanitarian reasons but were convinced it would lose them money. Instead, it restarted the field of transplantation. In Calne's initial human trials at Addenbrooke's Hospital in Cambridge in 1978, they found the drug could be toxic to human kidneys. But over time they adjusted the dose and found a safer level, and through the 1980s made further alterations that improved transplant outcomes even more.

It was by using these new drugs that Barnard's old rival, Norman Shumway, got the chance to have his own 'world first' – the first heart-lung transplant in 1981 performed with fellow surgeon Bruce Reitz. The recipient, Mary Gohlke, a forty-five-year-old woman whose heart and lungs had failed, asked her senator in Arizona to push the US Food and Drug Administration to allow Shumway's team permission to use the wonder drug cyclosporin. Permission was granted, and the two surgeons removed both her heart and her lungs. They described seeing Mary's 'totally empty chest' and wondering 'is this really going to work out?' Thanks to cyclosporin, it did, and Gohlke lived for five more years. The heart and lungs that Shumway and Reitz transplanted into her chest were still functioning up to the end – her autopsy five years later showed no evidence of rejection.[21]

Since this once-mysterious biological force has been identified and overcome, transplants have become routine miracles performed at hospitals around the world. In North

America, the UK and most other European countries, pathways to organs are highly regulated and governed by organizations such as the Human Tissue Authority. Organ shortages are now a chronic problem all over the world, however, and especially in countries where social security safety nets don't exist – or conflict has obliterated them – the situation is desperate. Poverty, disease and insecurity have brought dark echoes of the past, opportunities for greedy and unethical surgeons looking to profit as middlemen from the rich buying body parts from the poor.

Echoes of the Past

On the evening of 27 April 2007, citizens of Turkey turned on the news to see a shoot-out between the Istanbul police force and hospital guards at the private Sonmez Clinic. After a short stand-off, police swarmed through the building until they found a secret operating theatre. In the chaos, they discovered a clinical team, instruments in hand, about to conduct an illegal kidney transplant. They counted four patients. Two Arab-Israeli donors lay in green gowns, along with the two intended recipients. They – a South African and an Israeli – had each paid more than $200,000 for their bootleg body parts, their donors receiving just $10,000 apiece. Police wheeled the pale, cadaverous bodies out into the night along with a steady stream of scrubbed-up figures as the entire hospital staff was arrested. The chief surgeon and kingpin of the organization, Dr Yusuf Sonmez, was seen on Turkish TV, lab coat flapping as they frog-marched him to the police van. This was his fourth arrest.

Sonmez soon evaded his captors, was rearrested, then

sentenced to ten years' imprisonment. He was granted bail, which he skipped. Since then, he's been disappearing and reappearing all over the globe. In 2014 Serbian media reported that he had a house in Amsterdam and that someone had caught sight of him in South Africa. He'd also popped up in Kosovo in another high-profile case, and his wife let slip to Al Jazeera reporters that he was in Italy. Sonmez is still at large, on Interpol's wanted list for 'intentional infliction of grave injuries' and 'human trafficking', where the mugshot of this unassuming, bespectacled man takes its place amongst those of drug barons, rapists and murderers.[22]

We all know the state of organ transplants today – chronic shortage, increasing demand, lengthening waiting lists and poor quality of life hooked up to giant machines. Where legal donation satisfies only, at best, 10 per cent of demand, it's unavoidable that thousands of people will die waiting. Even in areas like Spain and the UK, where authorities have implemented 'presumed consent' and people have to opt *out* of organ donation instead of opting in, these problems have not gone away. There's some evidence, in fact, that even fewer organs get donated under this scheme. Although it's doubtless traumatic for a family, if a loved one actively opted to be on a donor register, their intention was clear. Under 'presumed consent', doctors still ask the family for permission to take organs, and if their son or daughter hadn't decided either way, families can't be sure what their loved ones actually wanted to happen. In their grief it's completely understandable that they sometimes refuse to let a 'procurement team' harvest the vital organs of their son or daughter. Given such poor odds, no wonder people look for alternatives, regardless of the law. When a South African studio released a film about this very impulse, *Bypass*, they created a website (newdayorgans.com) posing as a clinic offering organ procurement, complete with price list – R1,550,624 for a heart, R33,600 for a small intestine, and skin R140 per square cm. The film-makers say many tried to take up their offer in earnest.

On the other side of the market, donors rush to sell their organs to the highest bidder. One seventeen-year-old Syrian refugee told BBC reporters in 2017 that he had had no choice but to offer up one of his kidneys. His father and brother had been killed in the Syrian conflict, so the family had nothing to eat. Selling his organs looked like a way out. So, blindfolded and taken to a secret location, he was paid the equivalent of $8,000, which he used to pay the rent, clear his debt and support his mother and five sisters for a while. But now, with the money gone, in constant pain and with chronic exhaustion, he regrets his decision. The middleman in the transaction – a man called Abu Jaafer – has, meanwhile appeared on the BBC, bragging about being able to source and sell eyes, excusing his own involvement in human trafficking because he's 'helping people'.[23]

Given the dire consequences of unregulated and underground organ trading, it may appear that allowing the sale of certain organs like kidneys from live donors would be a good option. Recognizing and regulating a market would certainly help stop the theft of organs and could bring some accountability. The waiting lists, too, would plummet. This is what happened in Iran – the only country in the world where it's legal to sell your kidney and where waiting lists are now all but non-existent. Lari Zadeh, the president of the Kidney Transplant Association in Ahvaz, insists 'one kidney is enough for anyone'. But no one has yet studied the health of Iranian donors in any depth.[24]

Besides the unexamined health issue, assigning a financial

value to a body part has grave consequences. Life itself is given a value and traded, with thousands of people swindled out of their vital organs. In some cases, they're even stolen outright, as with an Indonesian maidservant who had her kidney removed at the behest of her Qatari employers. Not only did she not give consent for her organ to be removed, she didn't even know it had happened. Her employers told her she was going for a check-up. But she was anaesthetized and woke up in pain with an inexplicable scar. Not long after, her employers sent her back to Indonesia, discarding her as unfit to work. She only found out she was missing a kidney when she returned to her country and went to the doctor complaining of back pain.

The dystopian reality of body shopping has a dark precedent in teeth. Teeth snatching sounds like something from a sinister cartoon, a theft almost comical. It wasn't devastating in the same way or on the same scale as the organ trade, but it was still insidious: a symptom and cause of deep social inequality, a matter of the rich and powerful pressurizing the impecunious and marginalized. Henri Martinière was right in the seventeenth century when he said that men would cut one another's throats to preserve their lives. He foresaw the abuses of men like Sonmez and Jaafer, for whom the healthy poor are organ storage for the wealthy sick. And when a poor person becomes ill, there will be no hope for them. Lessons from the eighteenth century suggest that organ trafficking is linked to our familiar economic system, and to the modern ideas about consumerism that feed it. The uncomfortable truth is that those with more money have power over those with less.

7. Transplant Future

Transplantation seems always to have had two competing and compelling ideas connected to it. The first is that we are all unique. People throughout the ages, throughout the world, have leveraged transplants to retain their identity, to restore it, and even to give them a new identity altogether. A transplant coordinator in London told me a moving story about a terrified kidney recipient who received Christmas gifts each year addressed not to them but to their kidney. They were sent by the grief-stricken father of the donor. Though this is an extreme, tragic case, it nevertheless illustrates how difficult it can be to disassociate a person from their body. Whether it's a new nose, new tooth, new heart, or in the seventeenth century even a new set of humours, transplants have never been a simple matter of moving body parts around. They've always had consequences for people and their senses of self. That goes for the pioneering surgeons, perhaps, more than anyone, who have at times pursued transplant-related research with the conviction that it would make them or their patients immortal. If you could only transfer *younger* blood, you might become younger; if you could only replace your organs as they wore out, the human race would finally conquer death. Or so the idea goes.

The second big idea is more sobering and humbling, and almost the exact antithesis of the first: it seems that very little distinguishes us from one another. Human culture has largely evolved to convince us otherwise, but in truth you and I are made of the same stuff. Transplant surgeons have consistently shown us the many ways our bodies are compatible with one another, ranging from the inspiration skin-graft surgeons drew from plant grafts to the early scientists reimagining the human body as a machine. The machine metaphor has been particularly potent for organ-transplant surgeons, who in the twentieth century made good on this imagery, creating machines that outsourced our most sacred and vital functions to sausage skins and car parts.

But how can we be both unique *and* unremarkably similar? These two opposing ideas create a seemingly irresolvable tension, one that is particularly intensified with vascularized composite allotransplantation – the transplantation of entire body parts, like faces and hands.

It took surgeons until the end of the twentieth century to make allotransplantation a reality. It poses greater technical problems than the transplantation of internal organs and is far more complex than the relatively simple plumbing jobs required for the latter. It takes great skill, many hours and large multidisciplinary teams to make the connections of muscles, nerves, bones and skin necessary to transplant a functioning part. Rejection is a far more complex problem with these kinds of transplants, too. The man who received the first ever hand transplant, the New Zealander Clint Hallam, rejected it psychologically.

Hallam was in prison for fraud when he lost a hand in an accident with a circular saw in 1984. Fourteen years later, in 1998, he was being operated on in Lyon, which had been a century earlier host to Alexis Carrel's efforts to sew blood vessels together. The 1998 operation, led by Jean-Michel Dubernaud, lasted thirteen hours. In a news conference following the operation, Hallam talked about how he had to learn to use his new right hand from scratch, training a body that had been without one for fourteen years. It looked hopeful, but he soon started to resent his new hand and stopped taking the immunosuppression drugs. In 2001, he had it amputated. 'I am fully responsible for the rejection of this hand,' he said in an interview with the *New York Times*, 'which was satisfactory before I stopped my drugs.'[1] Though Hallam seems to have taken responsibility for the rejection, the psychologists Carla Bluhm and Nathan Clendenin have defended his decision, pointing out the difficulty of accepting the 'visual reality' of having someone else's hand. Hallam was framed as a 'bad patient', they say. If it wasn't for his criminal past, he might simply have said that the operation was 'creepy, or simply unwanted'.[2]

Accepting a hand seems to have equally dramatic effects. In India in 2016, an eighteen-year-old woman, Shreya Siddanagowder, lost her hands in a bus accident. The following year, a team of nearly forty worked over thirteen hours to graft new hands from a twenty-one-year-old male donor who died after crashing his bicycle. The man was slightly darker skinned, and over the next year and a half, as Siddanagowder had physical therapy to learn how to use her new hands, the skin gradually lightened to match her own skin tone. In a Facebook video in 2019, she said that she was the first woman in the world to have male hands, and those hands have since started to exhibit 'feminine features'. The mechanism behind these transformations is not yet clear, but it seems our relationship with our bodies is far more complicated than the popular spare-part model would suggest. Transplants are not as simple as fixing one part to another.[3]

Willem Kolff's old employer the Cleveland Clinic is also still at the forefront of transplant surgery. In 2008 the Polish surgeon Maria Siemionow performed the first near-complete face transplant there. Siemionow first transplanted rats' faces, calling one of her white recipients 'Zorro' because she'd given it a brown rat's face. In human patients, a face is an important functional part, without which you cannot breathe, bite, speak, smell, sip water from a cup, chew, or open your eyes – that is to say nothing of non-verbal communication. But a face is obviously far more than this. Siemionow likens the face to the heart – one of the organs to which we give an emotional weight,[4] and recognizes that, perhaps more than any other body part, our faces are what make us unique. Siemionow's work is incredibly important precisely because our faces are so caught up in our senses of self. At the same time, face transplants are possible only because scientists and surgeons have found the mechanisms that make body parts compatible with one another. Their close association with a person's identity might make us think of vascularized composite allotransplantation as fully embodying that tension between the two competing ideas at the heart of transplantation: we are unique, yet compatible.

The cutting edge of transplant research and biotechnology is taking this tension to breaking point. Possibilities have multiplied and expanded in recent years as bio-printing and stem-cell technology have matured. In the near future, this looks set to revolutionize transplantation. Eventually, hopefully, technology will move us away from needing donor organs at all. Then the need for powerful immunosuppression, expensive dialysis machines that grind life to a halt and organ waiting lists would all become things of the past. Being optimistic, technology might achieve all this more efficiently and ethically than encouraging more donation or legalizing the sale of organs.

Some medical professionals already use 3D printing.[5]

Models of body parts are reproduced from CAD files as cheap teaching tools, and surgeons can print precise scans of anatomy to familiarize themselves with complex cases before a major operation like separating conjoined twins. Printers can even produce simple mesh scaffolds – of a piece of skull, for example – that surgeons can implant directly into the body as part of reconstructive surgery.

One 3D-printed material, bioglass,[6] can be populated with stem cells and used to encourage bone growth as an alternative to titanium implants. The idea is that your stem cells, over time, will magically transform this material into bone – your own bone – so you regenerate what you, for instance, lost in a car accident, rather than have to rely on a non-organic implant. It takes a while for the bone to grow strong enough to hold any weight, so this is currently only used for applications like facial reconstruction.

It's also already possible to print human tissue directly as an ink made from a person's own cells. A biotech company in Vancouver, Aspect Biosystems, describes this process and their YouTube videos show entire printed body parts that, when placed into an incubator, come to life as cells connect with one another. Eventually, a printed windpipe or a heart valve can become an implantable part.

But the reality of printed hearts, ears, lungs, kidneys and so on is a long way off. Clinical trials are yet to take place, and the printers simply can't yet print at a high enough resolution to create most organic structures from scratch. Not that the printing technology is the greatest trial – it's a far bigger challenge to instal the body part and get the blood to flow around it so the recipient body adopts it. Still, the potential is awe-inspiring; it seems only a matter of time before technology will be precise enough to recreate the minute detail of vital organ anatomy, and work is under way to overcome the biological obstacles. According to colleagues at UCL in London, printing an entire replacement body part might only be a decade away.

In the meantime, bio-engineers are stripping existing structures of their cells by putting organs and other tissues into a bath of detergent. This is a process called decellularization. By dissolving cells, you are left with a collagen scaffold ready to be populated with cells from another organism. This solves the problem of printer resolution, at least, but it hasn't solved the concerns of animal rights activists – one potential solution is to take a pig's liver and turn it into a human one by depopulating its collagen frame and repopulating it with a particular patient's cells. A printed organ can be from another species. It doesn't, after all, have to look like that organ does when it forms in life. It just needs to do the same job.

The language such technologists use is horticultural: we grow, nurture, harvest and graft newly created parts. Scientists in the USA have even used decellularization technology

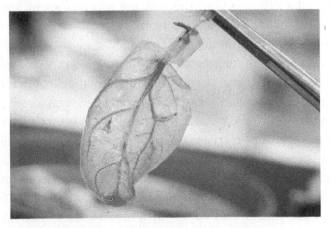

Figure 38 A spinach leaf seeded with heart cells.

to cross the boundaries of entire kingdoms. A couple of years ago, a team at Worcester Polytechnic Institute succeeded in decellularizing a spinach leaf and populating its scaffold with human heart tissue. All body parts need to have a vascular system – the networks of blood vessels that supply tissue with blood – if they are to be adopted by a host body. These complex and intricate structures already exist in nature, shared by organisms such as spinach – cheaper than pigs – so why not remove them from the vegetable kingdom and transplant them into the animal kingdom? Using a scaffold is another way to circumvent the need to print these structures. So, we could, in the future, also use plants as scaffolds in human bodies.[7] The same team is now working on populating spinach leaves with skin cells, which brings us back in a rather beautiful circle to the sixteenth century, when skin grafts were modelled on plant grafts.

Scientists in Japan have gone beyond even this and have successfully woven plant matter together with animal matter, grafting algae with rodent to create a hybrid animal-plant material. Cells united in this way are more efficient, say the team led by Yuji Haraguchi from Tokyo Women's Medical University. The animal cells produce carbon dioxide and ammonia, which the plant cells consume, and the plant cells produce the oxygen needed by the animal cells. Given the natural environment's carbon–nitrogen–oxygen cycles, the scientists say, their work is a recreation of everyday symbiotic relationships recreated on a cellular scale. One organism's waste product is recycled and used by the other. It's really an extension of the cycles we take advantage of all the time – we use animal matter in manure as a source of nitrogen for crops and plants, and we, in turn, breathe the oxygen products of plants.[8] To the scientists, the result is an efficient organic material. But if you can no longer tell the difference between the animal and the plant, you could also see it as a perversion of the distinctions that have helped us make sense of the world for thousands of years. To replace one organ with another is one thing, and still a contentious issue, but to create a hybrid organic matter on the cellular level is of another order entirely.

Transplant technology like this, operating on the cellular level, seems to be an extreme version of that aforementioned tension between our singularity and sameness. When we look so closely at human material on the cellular level, we cease to be people at all. The more intimately we examine our bodies, the less like individuals we become – a process that started as soon as we saw ourselves reflected in machines. When we look closer, we stop resembling ourselves not only as people, but also as animals. As the recognizable becomes unrecognizable, faces become noses which become skin which becomes cells. There must be a point at which we see the body as simply a combination of materials, and it even becomes hard to distinguish plant from animal anyway. At this level, zoomed in as far as can be, any kind of association with our identities simply disintegrates. We are already there: matter from algae and matter from mammals have already been joined into a single organism.

Some might protest about such transplant technology on religious or even humanitarian grounds, but perhaps our real problem with transplants – especially cross-species and cross-genus transplants – is the creeping realization that there is nothing intrinsically special about any one of us. Our body parts are, at least in principle, interchangeable, and if we are all the same, there is no reason for us to consider one person inherently superior to another. This, I think, is the real revolutionary idea always on the periphery, one I suspect we're not quite done with. And it's perhaps a fitting reflection for our inclusive and iconoclastic times.

In reality, of course, it is not that simple. Organ transplants currently require a lifelong commitment to a healthy lifestyle and a complicated regimen of drugs. There is a danger, too, when we see ourselves as separate to our bodies: an historical link with eugenics shows how recognizing the interchangeability of parts is not inevitably matched by egalitarian ideals. Thankfully, clinical transplantation is well regulated in much of the world. The profession is populated by compassionate and dedicated people, thanks to whom the sacrifices and wishes of donors are respected, and recipients are increasingly seen as part of the conversation, partners in their own care.

Still, what are we supposed to make of these great shifts on a cultural level? Though they may seem like a mere challenge to our taxonomies, the scale of the challenge is unprecedented and threatens to erase our very identity as humans. We're going to have to sacrifice some fundamental assumptions about ourselves, and that's monumental. But, as we've seen, similar boundaries have collapsed before. Most of us no longer think grafting skin will create a monster, and we've for the most part accepted that our personalities aren't transformed by a blood transfusion. It was once considered unnatural to cross gender boundaries – hermaphrodites were monsters. Perhaps it's immediately revolting to think about a being that is neither entirely plant nor animal, but as transplants develop in the future, could we also accept that this ancient plant/animal categorization might become an obsolete way of looking at life? The history – and future – of transplant surgery is tied up with these persistent questions about not only who we are, but also *what* we are, and what we might become.

Acknowledgements

My interest in the history of transplant surgery sprang from a photograph of a student, Jennifer Sutton, peering at her own heart through the glass of a museum case. This seemingly impossible situation came about in 2008 when, as a teenager, Sutton received a transplant as treatment for cardiomyopathy, a life-threatening condition that meant the walls of her heart had grown thicker than they were supposed to be. Just three months before the photograph was taken, she had donated her old heart to the Wellcome Collection in London, which arranged for it to be a special exhibit in its first public exhibition. 'Finally,' she told reporters as she gazed at the dead specimen with another person's heart beating away inside her, 'I can see this odd-looking lump of muscle that has given me so much upset.' The photographer captured both a touching story of a life saved and an implausible reality: a woman, with eyes full of life, staring at her own heart while her breath formed droplets on the outside of its case. I have never met Jennifer Sutton, but I have her to thank for the shivers her story sent up my spine, for helping me realize how transplant surgery goes beyond its image as a sterilized, scrubbed-up, hospital-bound affair.

I am most thankful for those at the centre of this book-writing process. *Spare Parts* would be far from publishable if it wasn't for the incredible Jenny Hewson, my agent, who took on and spent many hours with this project when it looked quite different. It was called *Dragon in a Suitcase* back then – an opaque title that my editors Assallah Tahir and

Juliet Annan saved me from having to explain every time I mentioned my book. To them, I am more grateful than I can express, for their immense contributions, commitment and support for me as an author. It has been a privilege to work and grow as a writer under their care, as it has to work with Trevor Horwood, whose detailed copy-editing improved this book immeasurably. Thank you, too, to Helen Garnons-Williams and all the staff at Fig Tree and Penguin Books.

The Wellcome Collection and Library, the British Library, UCL, Science Museum, Victoria and Albert Museum and Royal College of Surgeons have been constant sources of inspiration, as have the scores of people who have supported me in this project. James Peto, Sharon Messenger, Daniel Rees, Colin MacCabe, Laura Mulvey, Parveen Adams, Marco Daniel, Barry Curtis, Patrick Wright, Sharon Ruston, Tim Boon, Peter Morris all in one way or another shaped my early ideas. Phoebe Harkins and Ross MacFarlane deserve a special mention, as do Marta Ajmar and Heide Hatry. I am thankful, also, for the stimulating intellectual environment of the London Consortium, which is sadly now defunct, and especially Steven Connor, who spent more time and energy than anyone steering my early work. The late Mark Cousins was also a thought-provoking supervisor on the PhD project for a short period, as was Holly Tucker, whose work on seventeenth-century transfusion has helped me mould this narrative.

In my work on vascular anastomosis (sewing together blood vessels) I have drawn on the expertise of Fleur Oakes, who helped me formulate and put into words my thoughts on the significance of seeing the body as a textile or fabric. We met through Roger and Dusia Kneebone, whom I thank for a decade of inspirational talk and work. Roger also introduced me to the late John Wickham, and his wife, Ann, as well as the late Gunther Kress. I am sad that neither John nor Gunther will ever be able to read this book.

UCL's Department of Surgery and Interventional Sciences has also played an essential part in the making of this book. I particularly thank Barry Fuller. He is also responsible for my honorary position as Senior Research Associate at UCL. I am indebted, too, to the kidney-transplant pioneer Ossie Fernando and his son Bimbi, also a transplant surgeon, who, along with Barry, read through drafts of this work. As well as being a privilege to work with, they have both been valuable friends over the last decade or so. Thanks, too, to Clare Seldon, Chau Chong and Bern.

Thank you especially to Anna Harris for unparalleled support, inspiration and encouragement. And other colleagues in the Netherlands – Peter Peters, Bernike Pasveer, Karin Bijsterveld, Harro van Lente, Saskia Everts, Sven Dupré, Marjolijn Bol – have my sincerest gratitude for freely and generously giving their time to read through and discuss some of the ideas in this book.

The College of Physicians of Philadelphia Library very kindly offered me a Wood Institute Travel Grant, which enabled me to conduct a period of research in Philadelphia. I am indebted to Beth Lander, George Wohlreich and Robert Hicks there. Thank you particularly to Jacqui Bowman for making this and my various other visits to Philadelphia rewarding, and to Jeanene Johnson, who for a while – and for reasons beyond me – believed my name was 'Dr Crumpet'.

I extend a special thanks to Hayley Kruger at the Royal College of Surgeons in London for arranging for me to use the image of John Hunter's specimen P56. I thank, too, Joshua Gershlak and Glenn Gaudette for permission to use their 'spinach heart' leaf, and Hennie Joubert at the Heart of Cape Town Museum for his support.

It was a great encouragement to receive a special commendation for an early draft of this work from the Royal Society of Literature's Giles St Aubyn Award. It was a tremendous confidence boost at the right time of my writing career to have this acknowledgement. Thank you to Iain Sinclair, Laura Bates, Aida Edemariam and Fiona St Aubyn for judging my work to be worthy of praise. And to Molly Rosenberg and the staff at the RSL for all their exceptional work.

It remains to thank family and a few close personal friends for their support as I wrote this book. Matt Redman, Sally Marlow, Kelley Swain, Malcolm Creese, Eileen Dreyer, Martin Grant, Sharon Smithson, Remo Leonzi, Miranda Lowe York, Verena, and Eva Gersbach, and Karen and Fritz Reklah. Janice and Bill Rossen have shown unstinting support through all this project's various versions and drafts, and (Auntie) Shirley and (Uncle) Bill Tull have given more support than they know (including much of the contents of our home).

Finally, the greatest debt is to my grandparents, Mavis and James Little, and mother, Kim Craddock. And to my wife, Patricia Hammond, to whom this book is dedicated.

Notes

Prologue

1 Xiao-Ping Ren (2016), 'The Age of Head Transplants', *CNS Neuroscience & Therapeutics* 22(4): 257–9.
2 Cited in David Hamilton (2012), *A History of Organ Transplantation: Ancient Legends to Modern Practice*, Pittsburgh: University of Pittsburgh Press, p. 8.

1. Skin (1550–1597)

1 For more on the connection between historical skin grafting, identity and its dissolution: Paul Craddock (2012), 'Natural Material for Unnatural Ends', in Heide Hatry (ed.), *Not a Rose*, Milan: Charta.
2 G. Sperati (2009), 'Amputation of the Nose Throughout History', *Acta Otorhinolaryngologica Italica* 29(1): 44–50, p. 45.
3 Susan Redford (2002), *The Harem Conspiracy: The Murder of Ramesses III*, DeKalb: Northern Illinois University Press, pp. 7–11.
4 Sperati (2009), p. 48.
5 Maxwell Maltz (1946), *Evolution of Plastic Surgery*, New York: Froben Press, pp. 16–17.
6 Sperati (2009), p. 48.
7 Alan Clive Roberts (1971), *Facial Prostheses: The Restoration of Facial Defects by Prosthetic Means*, London: Kimpton.

8 John Robert Christianson (2003), *On Tycho's Island: Tycho Brahe, Science, and Culture in the Sixteenth Century*, Cambridge: Cambridge University Press, p. 173.

9 Megan Gannon (2012), 'Tycho Brahe Died from Pee, Not Poison', *LiveScience*: www.livescience.com/24835-astronomer-tycho-brahe-death.html.

10 Constance Head (1972), *Justinian II of Byzantium*, Madison: University of Wisconsin Press, pp. 24–100.

11 David Lindbergh (1978), *Science in the Middle Ages*, London: University of Chicago Press, p. 421.

12 Fioravanti's story is drawn from the following: William Eamon (1994), *Science and the Secrets of Nature*, Princeton: Princeton University Press; William Eamon (2010), *The Professor of Secrets: Mystery, Medicine and Alchemy in Renaissance Italy*, Washington, DC: National Geographic; Paolo Savoia (2017), 'Nature or Artifice? Grafting in Early Modern Surgery and Agronomy', *Journal of the History of Medicine and Allied Sciences* 72(1): 67–86; P. Santoni-Rugio and R. Mazzola (1997), 'Leonardo Fioravanti (1517–1588): A Barber-Surgeon Who Influenced the Development of Reconstructive Surgery', *Plastic and Reconstructive Surgery* 99(2): 570–75.

13 David O. Ross (1980), 'Non Sua Poma: Varro, Virgil and Grafting', *Illinois Classical Studies* 5: 63–71, p. 66.

14 George James Frazer (1911–15), *The Golden Bough: A Study in Magic and Religion* (12 vols.), London: Macmillan.

15 Pliny (1945), *Natural History, Volume IV: Books 12–16*, trans. H. Rackham, Cambridge, MA: Harvard University Press, p. 182.

16 A. G. Morton (1981), *History of Botanical Science*, London: Academic Press, p. 28.

17 Mark Grant (2000), *Galen on Food and Diet*, London: Routledge; Owen Powell (2002), *Galen on the Properties of Foodstuffs*, Cambridge: Cambridge University Press.

18 Manfred Horstmanshoff, Helen King and Claus Zittel (eds.) (2012), *Blood, Sweat and Tears: The Changing Concepts of Physiology from Antiquity into Early Modern Europe*, Leiden: Brill, p. 368.

19 Peter Wohlleben (2017), *The Hidden Life of Trees*, London: William Collins.

20 Fioravanti cited in Eamon (1994), p. 172.

21 Ibid., p. 171.

22 Leonardo Fioravanti (1561), *Il Capriccio Medicinale*, Venice: Ludovico Avanzo.

23 Eamon (1994), pp. 170–71.

24 Ibid., p. 187.

25 Ibid., p. 184.

26 Douglas Biow (2015), *On the Importance of Being an Individual in Renaissance Italy: Men, Their Professions and Their Beards*, Philadelphia: University of Pennsylvania Press, p. 137.

27 Ibid., p. 124.

28 Eamon (1994), p. 186.

29 Thomas Wright (2013), *Circulation: William Harvey's Revolutionary Idea*, London: Vintage, p. 34.

30 Philip Oldfield (2014), *Vesalius at 500: An Exhibition Commemorating the Five-Hundredth Anniversary of the Birth of Andreas Vesalius*, Toronto: University of Toronto Library, p. 16.

31 Grant (2000), p. 63.

32 Charles Hugh Talbot (1967), *Medicine in Medieval England*, London: Oldbourne, pp. 130–31.

33 Biow (2015), pp. 122–3.

34 Eamon (1994), p. 183.

35 Eamon (2010), pp. 7–9.

36 Otto L. Bettmann (1956), *A Pictorial History of Medicine*, Springfield: Charles C. Thomas, pp. 76–7, 108–11.

37 The story of Vesalius and Caius draws on the following sources: Oldfield (2014); Charles Donald O'Malley (1965),

English Medical Humanists: John Caius and Thomas Linacre, Lawrence: University of Kansas Press; Charles Donald O'Malley (1955), 'The Relations of John Caius with Andreas Vesalius and Some Incidental Remarks on the Giunta Galen and on Thomas Geminus', *Journal of the History of Medicine* 10(2): 147–72.

38 C. Galen (1916), *Galen on the Natural Faculties*, trans. John Brock, Cambridge, MA: Harvard University Press, pp. 141–2.

39 Julia Lyons (1998), 'Bloodletting in the Twentieth Century', unpublished dissertation, Wellcome Institute for the History of Medicine.

40 Quoted in Biow (2015), p. 137.

41 Steven Connor (2004), *The Book of Skin*, London: Reaktion, pp. 11–14.

42 Claudia Benthien (2002), *Skin: On the Cultural Border Between Self and the World*, New York: Columbia University Press, p. 64.

43 Eamon (2010), p. 99.

44 Ibid., pp. 55–6.

45 Biow (2015), pp. 140–42.

46 Eamon (1994), p. 186.

47 Eamon (2010), p. 99.

48 Ibid.

49 Raffi Gurunluoglu, Aslin Gurunluoglu and Jamie Arton (2017), 'Great Teachers of Gaspare Tagliacozzi (1546–1599)', *Journal of Medical Biography* 25(3): 161–9, p. 166.

50 Ibid., pp. 164–5.

51 Martha Teach Gnudi and Jerome Pierce Webster (1950), *The Life and Times of Gaspare Tagliacozzi, Surgeon of Bologna, 1545–1599*, New York: Herbert Reichner.

52 John Dixon Hunt (1996), *Garden and Grove*, Philadelphia: University of Pennsylvania Press, p. 44, note 24.

53 Claudia Lazzaro (1990), *The Italian Renaissance Garden: From the Conventions of Planting, Design, and Ornament to the Grand Gardens of Sixteenth-Century Central Italy*, New Haven: Yale University Press, p. 9, note 16.

54 Ibid., note 15.

55 Luke Morgan (2016), *The Monster in the Garden: Reframing Renaissance Landscape Design*, Philadelphia: University of Pennsylvania Press, p. 9.

56 Lazzaro (1990), p. 10.

57 Ibid., p. 8.

58 The story of Hermaphroditus I have taken from both the Penguin version of Ovid's *Metamorphoses* – Ovid (2004), *Metamorphoses: A New Verse Translation*, trans. David Raeburn, London: Penguin – and Ted Hughes's 2009 translation – *Tales from Ovid*, Oxford: Oxford University Press.

59 Morgan (2016), p. 12.

60 Lazzaro (1990), p. 8, note 3.

2. Blood, Animals to Animals (1624–1665)

1 Jaclyn Duffin (1999), *History of Medicine*, Toronto: University of Toronto Press, p. 171.

2 Frazer (1911–15), passim.

3 My chief sources for this section were: Andrew Gregory (2001), *Harvey's Heart: The Discovery of Blood Circulation*, Cambridge: Icon Books; William Harvey (1990), *The Circulation of the Blood and Other Writings*, trans. Kenneth J. Franklin, London: Dent; Douglas Starr (2000), *Blood: An Epic History of Medicine and Commerce*, New York: Alfred A. Knopf; Thomas Wright (2012), *Circulation: William Harvey's Revolutionary Idea*, London: Chatto and Windus.

4 Don Cameron Allen (1943), 'John Donne's Knowledge of Renaissance Medicine', *Journal of English and Germanic Philology* 42(3): 322–42; F. N. L. Poynter (1960), 'John Donne and William Harvey', *Journal of the History of Medicine and Allied Sciences* 15(3): 233–46, p. 235.

5 René Descartes (1649), *A Discourse on Method*, London: Printed by Thomas Newcombe, for John Holden at the Anchour in the new Exchange.

6 Marcello Malpighi (1661), *De Pulmonibus*, Bononiae: Typis Jo. Baptistae Ferronii.

7 Marcello Malpighi (1675), *Anatome Plantarum* . . . , London: Johannis Martyn; Domenico Bertoloni Meli (2011), *Mechanism, Experiment, Disease: Marcello Malpighi and Seventeenth-Century Anatomy*, Baltimore: Johns Hopkins University Press.

8 Colin Jones (2014), *The Smile Revolution in Eighteenth-Century Paris*, Oxford: Oxford University Press.

9 Wright (2012), p. 58.

10 John Aubrey (2016), Aubery's *Brief Lives*, ed. Oliver Lawson Dick, London: Vintage, p. 129.

11 Harvey (1990), p. 58.

12 Descartes (1649), p. 81.

13 Horstmanshoff, King and Zittel (2012), p. 385.

14 Aubrey (2016), p. 132.

15 Laurence Brockliss and Colin Jones (1997), *The Medical World of Early Modern France*, Oxford: Clarendon Press, p. 139.

16 Aubrey (2016), p. 128.

17 My chief source for Potter's story is Lisa Jardine (2003), *On a Grander Scale: The Outstanding Career of Sir Christopher Wren*, London: HarperCollins.

18 Francis Potter (1642), *Interpretation of the Number 666*, Oxford: Leonard Lichfield.

19 William Carleton Gibson (1970), 'The Biomedical Pursuits of Christopher Wren', *Medical History* 14(4): 331–41, p. 332.

20 Ovid (2004), p. 246.

21 Aubrey (2016), p. 248.

22 For Scarburgh and his circle, Christopher Wren and the formation of the Invisible College, I have relied on the following texts: Jardine (2003); Paul H. Hardacre (1956), *The Royalists During the Puritan Revolution*, The Hague: Martinus Nijhoff; J. J. Keevil (1952), 'Sir Charles Scarburgh', *Annals of Science* 8(2): 113–21; Charles Webster (1975), *The Great Instauration: Science, Medicine and Reform 1626–1660*, London: Duckworth; Barbara Shapiro and Robert G. Frank, Jr (eds.) (1979), *English Scientific Virtuosi in the 16th and 17th Centuries*, Los Angeles: William Andrews Clark Memorial Library, University of California.

23 Pete Moore (2003), *Blood and Justice*, Chichester: John Wiley, p. 39.

24 Ibid., p. 40.

25 Ibid., p. 42.

26 Starr (2000), pp. 11–12; Moore (2003), p. 70.

27 D'Arcy Power (1897), *William Harvey*, London: Longmans, Green, pp. 45, 122, 166–7.

28 Robert Boyle (1663), *Some Considerations Touching the Usefulness of Naturall Philosophy*, Oxford: Henry Hall, p. 64.

29 For the formation of the Royal Society: Jardine (2003).

30 Detailed in Moore (2003), pp. 47–52.

31 Frank Cole (1965), *Milestones in Anesthesia: Readings in the Development of Surgical Anesthesia, 1665–1940*, Lincoln: University of Nebraska Press, p. 7.

32 Anita Guerrini (1989), 'The Ethics of Animal Experimentation in Seventeenth-Century England', *Journal of the History of Ideas* 50(3): 391–407.

33 Ibid.

34 Robert G. Frank Jr (1980), *Harvey and the Oxford Physiologists*,
Berkeley, Los Angeles, London: University of California
Press, pp. 174–5; Francis Gotch (1908), *Two Oxford Physiolo-
gists: Richard Lower 1631–1691, John Mayow 1643–1679*, Oxford:
Clarendon Press, pp. 18–19.

35 'Tryals Proposed by Mr. Boyle to Dr. Lower . . . for the Improvement of Transfusing Blood Out of One Live Animal into
Another', *Philosophical Transactions*, 11 February 1666: 385–8.

3. Blood, Animals to Humans (1666–1670)

1 My sources for this section on transfusion in France are
Moore (2003); Starr (2000); Holly Tucker (2011), *Blood Work:
A Tale of Medicine and Murder in the Scientific Revolution*, New
York: W. W. Norton. I am especially indebted to Holly Tuck-
er's work; Tucker translated many of the French sources into
English for the first time and reconstructed many of these
scenes from archive material in her own book.

2 Cole (1965), p. 16.

3 Notes about Montmor, his rise and downfall, drawn from:
Tucker (2011); Jacques Roger (1992), *The Life Sciences in
Eighteenth-Century French Thought*, ed. Keith R. Benson, trans.
Robert Ellrich, Stanford: Stanford University Press; Albert
Van Helden (1974), 'The Telescope in the Seventeenth Cen-
tury', *Isis* 65(1): 38–58, p. 43; Roger Hahn (1971), *The Anatomy
of a Scientific Institution: The Paris Academy of Sciences, 1666–1803*,
Berkeley: University of California Press, p. 407.

4 *Journal des sçavans*, 8 April 1667: 96. Reprinted in *Philosophical
Transactions*, 10 February 1668: 617–24.

5 Tucker (2011), pp. 143–4.

6 Clarke to Oldenberg, April/May 1668, *Philosophical Transactions*, 18 May 1668: 672–82, cited in Tucker (2011), p. 149.

7 Moore (2003), p. 130.

8 My account of Coga's experiment draws on the following sources: Edmund King, 'An Account of the Experiment of Transfusion, Practised Upon a Man in London', *Philosophical Transactions*, 9 December 1667: 557–9; also with reference to Tucker (2011) and Moore (2003).

9 Details of Stubbe's reaction against transfusion taken from: Henry Stubbe (1670), *Legends no histories, or, A specimen of some animadversions upon The history of the Royal Society wherein, besides the several errors against common literature, sundry mistakes about the making of salt-petre and gun-powder are detected and rectified: whereunto are added two discourses, one of Pietro Sardi and another of Nicolas Tartaglia relating to that subject, translated out of Italian: with a brief account of those passages of the authors life . . . : together with the Plus ultra of Mr. Joseph Glanvill reduced to a non-plus, &c.*, London: n.p.

10 George Acton (1668), *Physical reflections upon a letter written by J. Denis, professor of philosophy and mathematicks, to Monsieur de Montmor, counsellor to the French King, and Master of Requests concerning a new way of curing sundry diseases by transfusion of blood*, London: T. R. for J. Martyn, pp. 8–9.

11 John Wilkins (1668), *An Essay towards a Real Character, and a Philosophical Language*, London: John Marttn [*sic*].

12 See Clive T. Probyn (1974), 'Swift and Linguistics: The Context Behind Lagado and Around the Fourth Voyage', *Neophilologus* 58: 425–39.

13 Thomas Shadwell (1676), *The Virtuoso. A Comedy*, London: T. N.

14 My main sources for Martinière's story are: Tucker (2011) and Starr (2000).

15 Additional details on Medea's story: Ovid (2004).

16 Mauroy's narrative relies heavily on the translations of French documents and archives made by Holly Tucker, and Tucker's own telling of the story (Tucker, 2011), Other sources include Moore (2003) and Starr (2000).

4. Teeth (1685–1803)

1 Charles Allen (1685), *The Operator for the Teeth: Shewing How to Preserve the Teeth and Gums for All the Accidents They are Subject To*, York: John White.
2 Hamilton (2012), p. 43.
3 Sidney Young (1890), *Annals of the Barber-Surgeons*, London: Blades, East and Blades, p. 178.
4 Christine Hillam (1991), *Brass Plate and Brazen Impudence*, Liverpool: Liverpool University Press, p. 117.
5 My main sources for this section: Mark Blackwell (2004), '"Extraneous Bodies": The Contagion of Live-Tooth Transplantation in Late-Eighteenth-Century England', *Eighteenth-Century Life* 28(1): 21–68; Paul Craddock (2018), 'Your Money Where Your Mouth Is: The Role of Consumerism in Eighteenth-Century Transplant Surgery', *History of Retailing and Consumption* 4(2): 1–15; Pierre Fauchard (1946), *The Surgeon Dentist, or, Treatise on the Teeth*, trans. Lillian Lindsay, London: Butterworth; Jones (2014); John R. Maestri (1989), 'Tooth Transplantation: An Idea Whose Time has Past [*sic*]', *Bulletin of the History of Dentistry* 37(2): 116; Henry W. Noble (2002), 'Tooth Transplantation: A Controversial Story', *History of Dentistry Research Group Newsletter* 11: 8–11.
6 B. R. Townend (1944), 'The Story of the Tooth-Worm', *Bulletin of the History of Medicine* 15(1): 37–58, pp. 43, 37.

7 Leo Kanner (1931), 'The Teeth of Gods, Saints, and Kings: Mythologies and Historical Contributions to Dental Folklore', *Medical Life* 38: 506–18, p. 517.

8 Malvin E. Ring (1985), *Dentistry: An Illustrated History*, New York: Harry N. Abrams, p. 28.

9 Details of the state of tooth care in France and of 'Le Grand Thomas' are drawn principally from Jones (2014).

10 Colin Jones (2000), 'Pulling Teeth in Eighteenth-Century Paris', *Past and Present* 166: 100–145, p. 134.

11 My section on Herman Boerhaave draws on the following sources: Andrew Cunningham (1990), 'Medicine to Calm the Mind: Boerhaave's Medical System, and Why it was Adopted in Edinburgh', in Andrew Cunningham and Roger French (eds.), *The Medical Enlightenment of the Eighteenth Century*, Cambridge: Cambridge University Press, pp. 40–66; Diana Faber (2007), 'Technological Metaphors and the Anatomy of Representations in Eighteenth-Century French Materialism and Dualist Mechanism', in Harry Whitaker, C. U. M. Smith and Stanley Finger (eds.), *Brain, Mind and Medicine*, New York: Springer, pp. 321–30; Peter J. Koehler (2007), 'Neuroscience in the Work of Boerhaave and Haller: Essays in Eighteenth-Century Neuroscience', in Whitaker, Smith and Finger, pp. 213–31; Peter Reill (2005), *Vitalizing Nature in the Enlightenment*, Berkeley: University of California Press; C. Schoneveld (1983), 'Samuel Johnson's *Life of Dr. Boerhaave* and a Dutch Translation', in J. van Dorsten (ed.), *The Age of Boerhaave*, Leiden: Brill, pp. 17–21.

12 Cunningham (1990), p. 47.

13 Faber (2007), p. 323.

14 My sources for the story of Vaucanson at the Hôtel de Longueville: Gaby Wood (2002), *Living Dolls: A Magical History*

of the Quest for Mechanical Life, London: Faber, p. 22. For additional mechanical details of Vaucanson's automata: Jacques Vaucanson (1742), *An Account of the Mechanism of an Automaton, or, Image Playing on the German Flute*, trans. J. T. Desaguliers, London: T. Parker, p. 13.

15 Wood (2002), pp. 24–6.

16 My section on Vaucanson's loom draws on Wood (2002), pp. 37–8.

17 Details of La Mettrie's assignation of sensation, memory, consciousness etc. as 'mechanical' are drawn from: Julien Offray de La Mettrie (1996), *Machine Man and Other Writings*, ed. and trans. Ann Thomson, Cambridge: Cambridge University Press; Aram Vartanian (1999), *Science and Humanism in the French Enlightenment*, Charlottesville: Rookwood Press; Charles T. Wolfe (2004), 'Epicuro-Cartesianism: La Mettrie's Materialist Transformation of Early Modern Philosophy', in Hartmut Hecht (ed.), *La Mettrie. Ansichte und Einsichte*, Berlin: Berlin Wissenschaftsverlag, pp. 75–96.

18 Erasmus Darwin (1804), *The Temple of Nature, or, the Origin of Society*, Baltimore: Bonsal & Niles, pp. 138–9.

19 Vartanian (1999), pp. 48, 56.

20 Coleridge (1796), 'On Doctors', from *Collected Letters of Samuel Taylor Coleridge*, ed. Earl Leslie Griggs, quoted in N. Vickers (2004), *Coleridge and the Doctors*, Oxford: Oxford University Press, p. 18.

21 For Trembley's story, I have drawn on the following sources: Marguerite Carozzi (1985), 'Bonnet, Spallanzani and Voltaire on Regeneration of Heads in Snails: A Continuation of the Spontaneous Generation Debate', *Gesnerus* 42: 265–88; Virginia P. Dawson (1987), *Nature's Enigma: The Problem of the Polyp in the Letters of Bonnet, Trembley and Réaumur*, Philadelphia: American Philosophical Society; Hamilton (2012).

22 For details about Bonnet and his earthworm see Carozzi (1985) and Dawson (1987).

23 E. L. M. Patrin (1788), *Zweifel gegen die Entwicklungstheorie*, trans. Georg Forster, Göttingen: Dieterich, pp. 97–119.

24 Cited in Aram Vartanian (1950), 'Trembley's Polyp, La Mettrie, and Eighteenth Century French Materialism', *Journal of the History of Ideas* 11(3): 259–86, p. 270.

25 Robert Whytt (1751), *Of the Motions of the Pupil and Muscles of the Internal Ear*, Edinburgh: Hamilton, Balfour and Neill.

26 Albrecht von Haller (1755), *A Dissertation on the Sensible and Irritable Parts of Animals*, London: Nourse.

27 Cited in William F. Bynum (1993), 'Cullen on the Nervous System', in A. Doig, J. P. S. Ferguson, I. A. Milne and R. Passmore (eds.), *William Cullen and the 18th Century Medical World*, Edinburgh: Edinburgh University Press, pp. 152–62; with further quotations from original letter: William Cullen (1784), 'A letter to Lord Cathcart, president of the Board of Police in Scotland: concerning the recovery of persons drowned, and seemingly dead', Edinburgh: C. Elliot.

28 Lester S. King (1974), 'George Cheyne, Mirror of Eighteenth Century Medicine', *Bulletin of the History of Medicine* 48(4): 517–39.

29 George Cheyne (1733), *The English Malady: or, A Treatise of Nervous Diseases of All Kinds*, London: G. Strahan, p. 105.

30 Thomas Trotter (1807), *A View of the Nervous Temperament*, London: Longman, Hurst, Rees and Orme, pp. xvii–xviii.

31 Thomas Aquinas (1975), *Summa Contra Gentiles, Book 4: Salvation*, Notre Dame: University of Notre Dame Press.

32 See Carole Reeves (ed.), (2010), *A Cultural History of the Human Body in the Enlightenment*, Oxford: Berg.

33 Jessica Riskin (2010), 'Medical Knowledge: The Adventure of Mr Machine, with Morals', in Reeves, pp. 73–92.

34 Barbara Wedgwood and Hensleigh Cecil Wedgwood (1980), *Wedgwood Circle 1730–1897: Four Generations of a Family and Their Friends*, London: Studio Vista.

35 Ruth Richardson (2010), 'Popular Beliefs About the Dead Body', in Reeves, p. 103.

36 Alun Withey (2015), *Technology, Self-Fashioning and Politeness in Eighteenth-Century Britain: Refined Bodies*, London: Palgrave.

37 See Craddock (2018) and Jones (2014).

38 Mayer Lewis (1772), *An Essay on the Formation, Structure, and Use of the Teeth*, London: J. Wheble, p. 23.

39 John Breval (1739), *The Art of Dress*, London: E. Curll.

40 Roger King (1998), *The Making of the Dentiste c.1650–1760*, Aldershot: Ashgate, p. 159.

41 Nicholas Dubois de Chemant (1797), *A Dissertation on Artificial Teeth in General*, London: J. Barker, p. 5.

42 James Bladen Ruspini (*c.*1802), *Observations on the Importance and Use of the Human Teeth*, London: Henry Reynell.

43 Roy Porter (1999), *The Greatest Benefit to Mankind: A Medical History of Humanity from Antiquity to the Present*, London: Fontana, p. 280.

44 David M. Knight (1998), *Science in the Romantic Era*, Aldershot: Ashgate, p. 19.

45 Wendy Moore (2006), *The Knife Man: Blood, Body-Snatching and the Birth of Modern Surgery*, London: Bantam Books, p. 37.

46 Details of Hume's cancer and consultation with Hunter are from the following sources: David Hume (1932), *The Letters of David Hume*, ed. J. Greig, Oxford: Clarendon Press, pp. 324–5; Roy Porter and Dorothy Porter (1989), *Patient's Progress: Doctors and Doctoring in Eighteenth-Century England*, Oxford: Polity in Association with Blackwell, p. 59; Ernest Campbell Mossner (2001), *The Life of David Hume*, Oxford: Oxford University Press, p. 595.

47 Moore (2006), p. 163.

48 Ibid., p. 174. This volume is also my main source for the story of Hunter's time in the army and with James Spence.

49 John Hunter (1771), *The Natural History of the Human Teeth: Explaining Their Structure, Use, Formation, Growth, and Diseases, Illustrated with Copper-Plates*, London: J. Johnson, p. 4.

50 Thomas Birch (1757), *History of the Royal Society of London for improving of natural knowledge, from its first rise*, London: A. Millar, pp. 315–16.

51 Henri-Louis Duhamel (1746), 'Recherches sur la réunion des plains des orbes et des Amimaux; et sur les greffes ou incisions, tant végétales qui'animales', *Compte Rendu De l'Académie Royale des Sciences*, 12 November 1746: 345–7.

52 Moore (2006), pp. 155–6.

53 Hunter's own account of the human–cockerel tooth transplant: Hunter (1778), p. 104.

54 For more on tooth transplantation and eighteenth-century literature, see Craddock (2018).

55 Anon (1757), *The Sedan, A Novel, etc.*, London: R. Baldwin.

56 John Hunter (1794), *A Treatise on the Blood, Inflammation, and Gun-Shot Wounds*, London: John Richardson and John Nicol.

57 Craddock (2018), p. 160.

58 Moore (2006), p. 222.

59 Ibid.

60 Bernhard Wolf Weinberger (1948), *An Introduction to the History of Dentistry*, St Louis: Mosby, p. 167.

61 The story of Anne Boulton's tooth transplant is related in her biography: Shena Mason (2005), *The Hardware Man's Daughter: Matthew Boulton and His 'Dear Girl'*, Chichester: Phillimore.

62 Mary Dorothy George (1937), *Catalogue of Political and Personal Satires, Preserved in the Department of Prints and Drawings in the British Museum*, vol. 6, London: British Museum.

63 Helenus Scott (1782), *Adventures of a Rupee*, Dublin: Messrs Price, pp. 189–91.

64 Francis Gentleman (1773), *The Pantheonites*, London: n.p.

65 Cited in Noble (2002), pp. 8–11.

66 Cited in Hamilton (2012), p. 46.

67 Cited in Ruth Richardson (1999), 'Transplanting Teeth: Reflections on Thomas Rowlandson's *Transplanting Teeth*', *The Lancet* 354(15): 1740.

68 Cited in Hamilton (2012), p. 47.

69 A. M. Mitscherlich (1815), 'The Replantation and Transplantation of Teeth', *Archives of Dentistry* 1: 169–84, p. 169.

70 Cited in Noble (2002).

71 Joseph Fox (1807), *The History and Treatment of the Diseases of the Teeth*, London: E. Cox.

72 J. F. Colyer (1919), *Dental Surgery and Pathology*: London: Longmans, Green.

73 Malvin E. Ring (1969), 'The Suffering Sewards', *Journal of the American Dental Association* 79(2): 233–4.

74 'Letter Regarding Skin Grafts', *The Gentleman's Magazine*, 9 October 1794, pp. 891–2.

75 Giuseppe Baronio (1985), *On Grafting in Animals: (Degli innesti animali)*, trans. Joan Bond Sax, Boston: Boston Medical Library; see also T. Gibson (1960), 'Flagellation and Free Grafting', *British Journal of Plastic Surgery* 13: 195–203, p. 197.

76 Joseph Constantine Carpue (1816), *An Account of Two Successful Operations for Restoring a Lost Nose from the Integuments of the Forehead, in the Case of Two Officers of His Majesty's Army: to which are prefixed, Historical and Physiological Remarks on the Nasal Operation; including Descriptions of the Indian and Italian Methods*, London: Hurst, Rees, Orme and Brown.

77 Hamilton (2012), p. 56.

78 For more on the debate between Abernethy and Lawrence and the continued relevance of vitalism in eighteenth-century culture, see: Sharon Ruston (2012), *Shelley and Vitality*, New York: Palgrave.

79 See Ruston's blog post for the British Library: www.bl.uk/ romantics-and-victorians/articles/the-science-of-life-and-death-in-mary-shelleys-frankenstein.

80 James Blundell (1818), 'Experiments on the Transfusion of Blood by the Syringe', *Medico-Chirurgical Transactions* 9(1): 56–92.

81 George McLoughlin (1959), 'The British Contribution to Blood Transfusion in the Nineteenth Century', *British Journal of Anaesthesiology* 31: 503–16, p. 503.

82 Blundell (1818), p. 75.

83 James Blundell (1825), *Researches Physiological and Pathological*, London: Cox, pp. 120–23.

84 James Blundell (1828), 'Observations on Transfusion of Blood', *The Lancet* 12(302): 321–4.

85 James Blundell (1834), *The Principles and Practice of Obstetricy: As at Present Taught by James Blundell*, London: Cox, pp. 142–3.

86 Ibid., pp. 72–3.

87 Harold W. Jones and Gulden Mackmull (1928), 'The Influence of James Blundell on the Development of Blood Transfusion', *Annals of Medical History* 10(5): 242–8.

5. Organs, Kidney (1901–1954)

1 C. Waller (1825), 'A Case of Haemorrhage from Inversion of the Uterus in Which the Operation of Transfusion Was Successfully Performed with Remarks on the Employment of Transfusion Generally', *Medico-Chirurgical Transactions* 35: 413–35.

2 Kim Pelis (2001), 'Blood Standards and Failed Fluids: Clinic, Lab, and Transfusion Solutions in London, 1868–1916', *History of Science* 39: 185–213.

3 McLoughlin (1959), p. 515.

4 Details of Landsteiner's discovery from: Paul Speiser (1975), *Karl Landsteiner, the Discoverer of the Blood-Groups and a Pioneer in the Field of Immunology*, trans. Richard Rickett, Vienna: Hollinek; Hans Peter Schwarz and Friedrich Dorner (2003), 'Karl Landsteiner and His Major Contributions to Haematology', *British Journal of Haematology* 121(4): 556–65.

5 My sources for the story of Carnot's assassination are the following: Anon. (1894), 'Caserio Struggled for Life; the Assassin's Courage Failed Him in the End', *New York Times*, 16 August, p. 5; David Hamilton (2017), *The First Transplant Surgeon: The Flawed Genius of Nobel Prize Winner, Alexis Carrel*, Hackensack: World Scientific Publishing, p. 12; Nicholas L. Tilney (2003), *Transplant: From Myth to Reality*, New Haven: Yale University Press, p. 36.

6 Robert Cusimano, Michael Cusimano and Steven Cusimano (1984), 'The Genius of Alexis Carrel', *Canadian Medical Association Journal* 131(9): 1142–50; Steven G. Friedman (2015), 'The End-to-End Anastomosis of John B. Murphy', *Journal of Vascular Surgery* 62(2): 515–17, p. 517.

7 Sheldon Marvin Levin (2015), 'Alexis Carrel's Historic Leap of Faith', *Journal of Vascular Surgery* 61(3): 832–3.

8 Hamilton (2017), p. 21.

9 My own recent work with Fleur Oakes reconstructs both Carrel's technique of vascular anastomosis (sewing together blood vessels) along with Leroudier's technique. For more information, see Paul Craddock (2021), 'The Cigarette Paper, the Embroiderer, and the Gendered Craft of Vascular Surgery', in Anna Harris and John Nott (eds.), *Between Blackboards*

and Formaldehyde: Matters of Medical Knowledge, Bristol: Intellect, in press.

10 For example Harold Ellis (2019), 'The Story of Peripheral Vascular Surgery', *Journal of Perioperative Practice* 29(8): 245–56, p. 256; Roger Kneebone, Fleur Oakes and Colin Bicknell (2019), 'Reframing Surgical Simulation: The Textile Body as Metaphor', *The Lancet* 393(10166): 22–3, p. 23.

11 I am indebted to Oakes's knowledge and experience as a three-dimensional embroiderer, and our sustained collaboration together with Professor Roger Kneebone at Imperial College London. For more about Kneebone's expertise on experts like Oakes, see his 2020 *Expert: Understanding the Path to Mastery*, London: Penguin.

12 Craddock (2020).

13 Alexis Carrel (1902), 'La technique opératoire des anastomoses vasculaire et la transplantation des viscères', *Lyon Médical* 99: 859–62.

14 Cited in Hamilton (2017), p. 22.

15 Ibid.

16 On Carrel at Lourdes, see ibid., pp. 23–4.

17 Joseph T. Durkin (1965), *Hope for Our Time: Alexis Carrel on Man and Society*, New York: Harper and Row.

18 Tilney (2003), pp. 40–41.

19 For more details on the Cosmas and Damian myth and its countless variations and depictions, see Kees Zimmerman (ed.) (2013), *One Leg in the Grave Revisited: The Miracle of the Transplantation of the Black Leg by the Saints Cosmas and Damian*, Groningen: Barkhuis, pp. 12–14.

20 For an interpretation of the significance of race and identity in the story, see: Jean E. Feerick (2010), *Strangers in Blood: Relocating Race in the Renaissance*, Toronto: University of Toronto Press, p. 10.

21 This part of Carrel's life and the development of vascular anastomosis with Guthrie has been thoroughly reconstructed and researched by David Hamilton in Hamilton (2017).

22 My main sources for the story of Mary Lambert are: Hamilton (2017), pp. 105–7; Samuel W. Lambert (1908), 'Melaena Neonatorum with Report of a Case Cured by Transfusion', *Medical Record* 73: 885–7; J. G. Walker (1973), 'Carrel's Transfusion of a Five Day Old Infant', *Surgery, Gynecology & Obstetrics* 137: 494–6.

23 See John H. Barker, Johannes M. Frank and Liudmila Leppik (2015), 'Head Transplantation: Editorial Commentary', *CNS Neuroscience and Therapeutics* 21(8): 613–14.

24 Cited in Tilney (2003), p. 93.

25 Ibid.

26 My source for Brinkley: Pope Brock (2008), *Charlatan: America's Most Dangerous Huckster, the Man Who Pursued Him, and the Age of Flimflam*, New York: Crown Publishing Group.

27 My source for Voronoff: Petar Bajic, Steven H. Selman and Michael A. Rees (2012), 'Voronoff to Virion: 1920s Testis Transplantation and AIDS', *Xenotransplantation* 19(6): 337–41.

28 For this entire 'Immortality' section, I have relied primarily on David Friedman (2008), *The Immortalists: Charles Lindbergh, Dr. Alexis Carrel, and Their Daring Quest to Live Forever*, New York: Harper Perennial. Friedman originally reconstructed many of the events regarding Carrel and Lindbergh and their quest for immortality. Also Hamilton (2017), pp. 379–89.

29 Hamilton (2017), p. 430.

30 My main source for Demikhov's narrative is Hamilton (2012), pp. 199–209.

31 Details of Brukhonenko: Igor E. Konstantinov (2000), 'Sergei S. Brukhonenko: The Development of the First Heart-Lung

Machine for Total Body Perfusion', *Annals of Thoracic Surgery* 69(3): 962–6.

32 Hamilton (2017), pp. 67–8.

33 https://archive.org/details/0226_Experiments_in_the_ Revival_of_Organisms_20_36_46_00.

34 My main source for Willem Kolff's story is Kolff's biography: Paul Heiney (2002), *The Nuts and Bolts of Life: Willem Kolff and the Invention of the Kidney Machine*, Thrupp: Sutton Publishing. Additional sources: Tilney (2003), pp. 144–7; Joshua D. Mezrich (2019), *When Death Becomes Life: Notes from a Transplant Surgeon*, New York: HarperCollins.

35 My main source for Medawar's story is his autobiography: Peter Medawar (1986), *Memoir of a Thinking Radish*, Oxford: Oxford University Press. Further source: Mezrich (2019), pp. 60–66.

36 Sources for this section about Hume and Hufnagel's kidney transplant: Roy Calne (1998), *The Ultimate Gift: The Story of Britain's Premier Transplant Surgeon*, London: Headline; Hamilton (2012); Francis D. Moore (1995), *A Miracle and a Privilege: Recounting a Half Century of Surgical Advance*, Washington, DC: Joseph Henry Press; Joseph E. Murray (2001), *Surgery of the Soul: Reflections on a Curious Career*, Boston: Boston Medical Library; Tilney (2003).

6. Organs, Heart (1967–)

1 My main source for Kolff's story in this section: Heiney (2003).

2 My main sources for the race to transplant a human heart are: Christiaan Barnard and Curtis Bill Pepper (1970), *Christiaan Barnard: One Life*, London: Harrap; Hamilton (2012); Donald McRae (2006), *Every Second Counts: The Race to Transplant the*

First Human Heart, New York: G. P. Putnam's Sons; Mezrich (2019); Moore (1995); Tilney (2003).

3 Barnard and Pepper (1970), pp. 183–4.

4 Norman E. Shumway cited in René Küss and Pierre Bourget (1992), *An Illustrated History of Organ Transplantation*, Rueil-Malmaison: Laboratoires Sandoz, p. 113.

5 Barnard and Pepper (1970), pp. 329–30.

6 Moore (1995), p. 177.

7 My main source for Calne's story, 6MP and cyclosporin: Calne (1998) and Moore (1995).

8 Calne (1998), p. 49.

9 Murray (2001), p. 117.

10 Richard R. Lower, Eugene Dong and Norman E. Shumway (1965), 'Suppression of Rejection Crises in the Cardiac Homograft', *Annals of Thoracic Surgery* 1(5): 645–9, p. 645.

11 For this section on Denise Darvall and Louis Washkansky, my main sources were: Barnard and Pepper (1970), Hamilton (2012), McRae (2006), Mezrich (2019) and Tilney (2003).

12 Barnard and Pepper (1970), p. 280.

13 Shumway's colleague James Hardy quoted in McRae (2006), p. 208.

14 Ibid., p. 212.

15 Barnard and Pepper (1970), pp. 392–3.

16 Mezrich (2019), p. 155.

17 Ibid., pp. 152–5.

18 Calne (1998), p. 128.

19 Donald Longmore (1968), *Spare-Part Surgery: The Surgical Practice of the Future*, London: Aldus Books.

20 My source for this section on cyclosporin is Calne's own account: Calne (1998), pp. 115–21.

21 Mezrich (2019), pp. 160–61.

22 www.aljazeera.com/indepth/features/2015/10/kidney-worlds-biggest-organ-market-151007074725022.html.

23 www.bbc.co.uk/news/magazine-39272511.

24 www.theguardian.com/society/2015/may/10/kidneys-for-sale-organ-donation-iran.

7. Transplant Future

1 Maria Siemionow (2019), *Face to Face: A Short History of Face Transplantation*, Cham: Springer, p. 43.

2 Carla Bluhm and Nathan Clendenin (2009), *Someone Else's Face in the Mirror: Identity and the New Science of Face Transplants*, Westport: Praeger, p. 16.

3 www.livescience.com/hand-transplant-skin-lighten.html.

4 Siemionow (2019), p. 4.

5 https://3dprint.com/163831/3d-printing-the-future-of-surgery/.

6 www.bbc.co.uk/programmes/b08rq6dl.

7 Joshua R. Gershlak et al. (2017), 'Crossing Kingdoms: Using Decellularized Plants as Perfusable Tissue Engineering Scaffolds', *Biomaterials* 125: 13–22.

8 Yuta Okamoto et al. (2019), 'Mammalian Cell Cultivation Using Nutrients Extracted from Microalgae', *Biotechnology Progress* 36(2); Yuji Haraguchi et al. (2017), 'Thicker Three-Dimensional Tissue from a "Symbiotic Recycling System" Combining Mammalian Cells and Algae', *Scientific Reports* 7(1): 41594.

Selected Bibliography

Sixteenth Century

Biow, Douglas (2015). *On the Importance of Being an Individual in Renaissance Italy: Men, Their Professions and Their Beards*. Philadelphia: University of Pennsylvania Press.

Connor, Steven (2004). *The Book of Skin*. London: Reaktion.

Eamon, William (1994). *Science and the Secrets of Nature*. Princeton: Princeton University Press.

———— (2010). *The Professor of Secrets: Mystery, Medicine and Alchemy in Renaissance Italy*. Washington, DC: National Geographic.

Grant, Mark (2000). *Galen on Food and Diet*. London: Routledge.

Maltz, Maxwell (1946). *Evolution of Plastic Surgery*. New York: Froben Press.

Oldfield, Philip (2014). *Vesalius at 500: An Exhibition Commemorating the Five-Hundredth Anniversary of the Birth of Andreas Vesalius*. Toronto: University of Toronto Library.

Seventeenth Century

Aubrey, John (2016). Aubrey's *Brief Lives*, ed. Oliver Lawson Dick. London: Vintage.

Brockliss, Laurence, and Jones, Colin (1997). *The Medical World of Early Modern France*. Oxford: Clarendon Press.

Frank, Robert G., Jr (1980). *Harvey and the Oxford Physiologists*. Berkeley, Los Angeles, London: University of California Press.

Gregory, Andrew (2001). *Harvey's Heart: The Discovery of Blood Circulation*. Cambridge: Icon Books.

Jardine, Lisa (2003). *On a Grander Scale: The Outstanding Career of Sir Christopher Wren*. London: HarperCollins.

Moore, Pete (2003). *Blood and Justice*. Chichester: John Wiley.

Starr, Douglas (2000). *Blood: An Epic History of Medicine and Commerce*. New York: Alfred A. Knopf.

Tucker, Holly (2011). *Blood Work: A Tale of Medicine and Murder in the Scientific Revolution*. New York: W. W. Norton.

Wright, Thomas (2012). *Circulation: William Harvey's Revolutionary Idea*. London: Chatto and Windus.

Eighteenth and Nineteenth Centuries

Hillam, Christine (1991). *Brass Plate and Brazen Impudence*. Liverpool: Liverpool University Press.

Jones, Colin (2014). *The Smile Revolution in Eighteenth-Century Paris*. Oxford: Oxford University Press.

King, Roger (1998). *The Making of the Dentiste c. 1650–1760*. Aldershot: Ashgate.

Knight, David M. (1998). *Science in the Romantic Era*. Aldershot: Ashgate.

La Mettrie, Julien Offray de (1996). *Machine Man and Other Writings*, ed. and trans. Ann Thomson, Cambridge: Cambridge University Press.

Mason, Shena (2005). *The Hardware Man's Daughter: Matthew Boulton and His 'Dear Girl'*. Chichester: Phillimore.

Moore, Wendy (2006). *The Knife Man: Blood, Body-Snatching and the Birth of Modern Surgery*. London: Bantam Books.

Reeves, Carole (ed.) (2010). *A Cultural History of the Human Body in the Enlightenment*. Oxford: Berg.

Reill, Peter (2005). *Vitalizing Nature in the Enlightenment*. Berkeley: University of California Press.

Ring, Malvin E. (1985). *Dentistry: An Illustrated History*. New York: Harry N. Abrams.

Withey, Alun (2015). *Technology, Self-Fashioning and Politeness in Eighteenth-Century Britain: Refined Bodies*. London: Palgrave.

Wood, Gaby (2002). *Living Dolls: A Magical History of the Quest for Mechanical Life*. London: Faber.

Twentieth and Twenty-First Centuries

Barnard, Christiaan, and Pepper, Curtis Bill (1970). *Christiaan Barnard: One Life*. London: Harrap.

Brock, Pope (2008). *Charlatan: America's Most Dangerous Huckster, the Man Who Pursued Him, and the Age of Flimflam*. New York: Crown Publishing Group.

Calne, Roy (1998). *The Ultimate Gift: The Story of Britain's Premier Transplant Surgeon*. London: Headline.

Friedman, David (2008). *The Immortalists: Charles Lindbergh, Dr. Alexis Carrel, and Their Daring Quest to Live Forever*. New York: Harper Perennial.

Hamilton, David (2012). *A History of Organ Transplantation: Ancient Legends to Modern Practice*. Pittsburgh: University of Pittsburgh Press.

―――― (2017). *The First Transplant Surgeon: The Flawed Genius of Nobel Prize Winner, Alexis Carrel*. Hackensack: World Scientific Publishing.

Heiney, Paul (2002). *The Nuts and Bolts of Life: Willem Kolff and the Invention of the Kidney Machine*. Thrupp: Sutton Publishing.

Longmore, Donald. (1968). *Spare-Part Surgery: The Surgical Practice of the Future*. London: Aldus Books.

McRae, Donald (2006). *Every Second Counts: The Race to Transplant the First Human Heart*. New York: G. P. Putnam's Sons.

Medawar, Peter (1986). *Memoir of a Thinking Radish*. Oxford: Oxford University Press.

Mezrich, Joshua D. (2019). *When Death Becomes Life: Notes from a Transplant Surgeon*. New York: HarperCollins.

Moore, Francis D. (1995). *A Miracle and a Privilege: Recounting a Half Century of Surgical Advance*. Washington, DC: Joseph Henry Press.

Murray, Joseph E. (2001). *Surgery of the Soul: Reflections on a Curious Career*. Boston: Boston Medical Library.

Siemionow, Maria (2019). *Face to Face: A Short History of Face Transplantation*. Cham: Springer.

Tilney, Nicholas L. (2003). *Transplant: From Myth to Reality*. New Haven: Yale University Press.

Index

Page references in *italics* indicate images.

blood:
circulation system, Harvey discovers
6, 50–59, *54*, 60, 63, 64–5, 67, 68,
69–70, 71, 79–80, 82, 90, 92, 95,
126, 134
humoralism and *29*, 30–31, 37, 80,
89, 90, 96, 125, 156
'vital principle' in 27, 59, 156–7,
166–70, *168*, *169*
blood bank 203–4, 211
bloodletting *29*, 30–31, 37, 80, 89, 90,
96, 156
blood serum 172, 191, 192
blood transfusion 6, 49–115, 126,
144–5, 167–70, 171, 230
abandoned, nineteenth-century 114
blood types, discovery of and 6,
172–6, 187, 217
Blundell and 7, 167–70, *168*, *169*
Boyle's experiments 67–9, 70, 71,
72, 74, 75, 76–7, 87, 101, 126
Coga transfusion 96–8, 108
cultural weight of blood and 57–8
Denis and 70, 80–83, 86–8, 89–95,
97, 101, 102–3, 105, 106, 108,
109, 116
donor–recipient relationship,
first 73
earliest references to 49–50
essential role in modern transplant
surgery 50, 114–15
first blood transfusion 59–77,
78–88
Harvey's discovery of circulation of
blood and 6, 50–59, *54*, 60, 63,
64–5, 67, 68, 69–70, 71, 79–80, 82,
90, 92, 95, 126, 134
human blood compatible with only
human bodies concept
established 170

human-to-human transfusions in
order to save a life, first 7, 170
Italian blood transfusion (1668)
111
Jason and the Argonauts and
60–62, 63, 107
Lower's experiments 72–7, *75*,
78, 82, 83, 91, 92, 93, 94,
95, 96–9, 101, 102, 108,
114–15
madness and 96–8, 108–14
Martinière opposition to 101–8,
113, 114, 162, 249
Mauroy transfusion 108–14
popular attitudes towards
100–101
Perrault experiments 78–80, 81, 86,
87, 91, 113
personality/identity and 105–6,
110, 144–5, 258
Potter experiments 60, 61, 62, 63–4,
71, 72, 73, 76, 79, 93
substitution of blood as alternative
to 171
tooth transplantation and 7,
167–70, *168*, *169*
vascular anastomosis technique and
173–85, *178*, 189, 190, 251
'vital principle' in the blood
concept/vitalism and 27, 59,
156–7, 166–70, *168*, *169*, 171
vivisection, justifications for and
74–6
Wilkins experiments 67, 68, 69, 71,
96, 98, 100
Wren experiments 66, 67, 68, 69,
70–71, 72, 73, 78, 93, 100, 101
xeno-transfusion (animals to
humans), first *88*, 89–114,
99, *111*

He just wanted a decent book to read ...

Not too much to ask, is it? It was in 1935 when Allen Lane, Managing Director of Bodley Head Publishers, stood on a platform at Exeter railway station looking for something good to read on his journey back to London. His choice was limited to popular magazines and poor-quality paperbacks – the same choice faced every day by the vast majority of readers, few of whom could afford hardbacks. Lane's disappointment and subsequent anger at the range of books generally available led him to found a company – and change the world.

'We believed in the existence in this country of a vast reading public for intelligent books at a low price, and staked everything on it'
Sir Allen Lane, 1902–1970, founder of Penguin Books

The quality paperback had arrived – and not just in bookshops. Lane was adamant that his Penguins should appear in chain stores and tobacconists, and should cost no more than a packet of cigarettes.

Reading habits (and cigarette prices) have changed since 1935, but Penguin still believes in publishing the best books for everybody to enjoy. We still believe that good design costs no more than bad design, and we still believe that quality books published passionately and responsibly make the world a better place.

So wherever you see the little bird – whether it's on a piece of prize-winning literary fiction or a celebrity autobiography, political tour de force or historical masterpiece, a serial-killer thriller, reference book, world classic or a piece of pure escapism – you can bet that it represents the very best that the genre has to offer.

Whatever you like to read – trust Penguin.